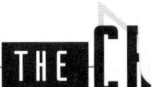 

# THE WORKAHOLIC'S WORKOUT

## CRUNCH

HATHERLEIGH

NEW YORK

Getfitnow.com Books
An Independent Imprint of Hatherleigh Press

Copyright © 2000 by Crunch Fitness

All rights reserved. No part of this book may be reproduced in any form or by any means, electronic or mechanical, including photocopying, recording, or by any information storage or retrieval system, without permission in writing from the publisher.

Getfitnow.com Books
An Independent Imprint of Hatherleigh Press
an affiliate of W.W. Norton & Company
500 Fifth Avenue
New York, NY 10110
1-800-367-2550
www.getfitnow.com

Before beginning any strenuous exercise program consult your physician. The author and publisher of this book and workout disclaim any liability, personal or professional, resulting from the misapplication of any of the training procedures described in this publication.

All GetFitNow.com books are available for bulk purchase, special promotions, and premiums. For more information, please contact the manager of our Special Sales department at 1-800-367-2550.

Library of Congress Cataloging in-Publication Data

Crunch Fitness,
    Workouts for workaholics / Crunch.
       p.    cm. — (The Crunch Fitness Series)
    Includes bibliographical references
    ISBN 1-57826-041-8 (alk. paper)
    1. Workaholics—Health and hygiene.  2. Exercise.  3. Stress management.
4. Physical fitness   I. Crunch.  II. Series.
RA781.W67  2000
613.7'1—dc21                                                   99-087622
                                                                                                         CIP

Series Editor: Heather Ogilvie
Cover design: Lisa Fyfe
Text design and composition: John Reinhardt Book Design
Photographs: Chia Messina

Printed in Canada on acid-free paper

10  9  8  7  6  5  4  3  2  1

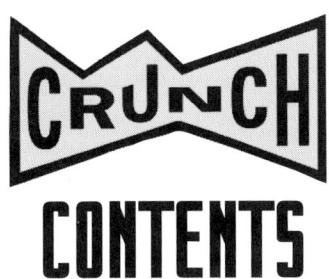

# CONTENTS

Introduction to Crunch Fitness Guides ................................................. v
About the Authors ................................................................................ vii

### PART 1
Step 1: Admitting You're a Workaholic — 1

### PART 2
Step 2: Working in the Workout — 7

### PART 3
Step 3: Learning How to Relax — 41

### PART 4
Step 4: Eating Well — 55

### PART 3
Step 5: Combating Stress — 69

Appendix A: Further Reading ............................................................. 79
Appendix B: Advanced Workout ........................................................ 81
Crunch Locations ................................................................................ 83

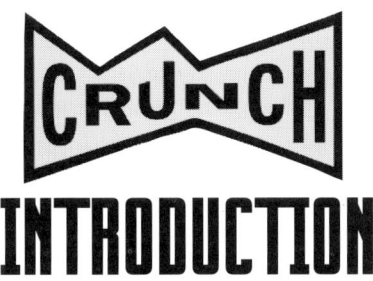

# INTRODUCTION

Welcome to CRUNCH! For over a decade, we've been welcoming people of all shapes, sizes, ages, and fitness levels to our gyms. As we've expanded from a tiny, one-room aerobics studio in New York's East Village to cities across the country (and even to Tokyo), we've offered group fitness classes, personal training, and equipment to appeal to everyone from stressed-out workaholics and jet setters to senior citizens and expectant moms. We're living up to our motto, "No Judgements!"

We're aware that some people shy away from joining a gym or from starting a fitness program because they think it demands too great a change in their lifestyle. But at CRUNCH, we believe you shouldn't have to change your lifestyle in order to be fit. In fact, we believe your workout should change to fit your lifestyle. It is our firm belief that the success of a fitness program has nothing to do with how many hours you spend in the gym, but how good you feel when you're outside the gym, living your life.

That's why we've created these guides—to show you that no matter what your lifestyle, there's a workout you can do that will complement it and get you fit. For example, we designed the *Road Warrior Workout* for people who spend a lot of time traveling on business. These folks don't have to give up their fitness programs—in fact, by doing a workout specially adapted to life on the road, they can maintain their fitness level and become less susceptible to all the common aches and discomforts of travel.

*Get Fit in a CRUNCH* is for those people who are trying to shape up in time for a big event—a wedding, a reunion, a trip to the beach. Based on CRUNCH's popular class, Emergency Beach Training, *Get Fit in a CRUNCH* lays out a safe, effective four-week workout, 12-week workout, and six-month workout.

# INTRODUCTION

Since the hardest part of any fitness program is starting it, we've written *Beginner's Luck* to help people stay motivated and become more familiar with—and less intimidated by—basic cardiovascular and strength training exercises. It's a workout you can take at your own pace, according to your own goals.

Other CRUNCH guides include *The Workaholic's Workout*, targeting time-pressed workaholics; *On Your Mark. Get Set. Go! Marathon Training*, for first-time marathon runners; and *Posture Perfect*, for people who want to eliminate or avoid common back pain and improve posture.

At CRUNCH, we don't want you to conform to some workout fad or a lifestyle of spending more time at the gym than at play. We want to give you workout options that will conform to your lifestyle—without judgement.

**Doug Levine**
*Founder and CEO*
*Crunch Fitness International, Inc.*
*www.crunch.com*

# ABOUT THE AUTHORS

**Charlie Morris**, a trainer in CRUNCH's Atlanta gyms, designed the Workaholic's Workout. Having trained workaholics for years, Charlie has been interviewed about his unique workout in the magazines *Elle* and *Women's Health*, and on the TV show, *Peachtree Morning*. Post-rehab, ISSA, and stretch certified, Charlie's background includes judo, wrestling, and kickboxing.

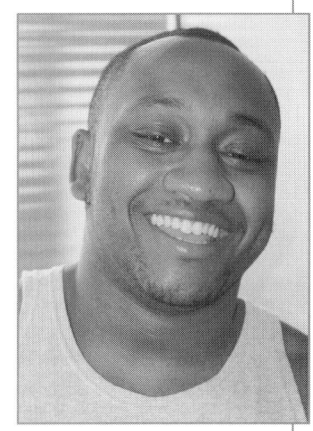

**Amy Ippoliti** contributed the relaxing and energizing yoga poses described in Chapter 3. A devoted student of yoga for 13 years, Amy is a certified Vinyasa yoga instructor and an affiliated Anusara yoga instructor. Her teaching arises from her dedicated studies at Om Yoga Center in Anusara yoga with John Friend and from her background as an ACE-certified fitness trainer. Amy teaches throughout Manhattan privately, in corporations, and at CRUNCH Fitness, Om Yoga Center, and Kimball Studio.

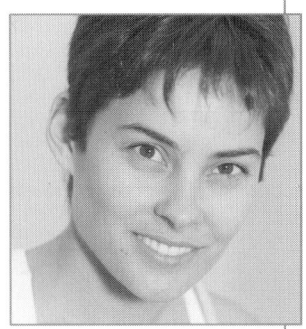

## ABOUT THE AUTHORS

**Larry Krug** and **Jennifer Nardini** designed the nutritional program in Part 4.

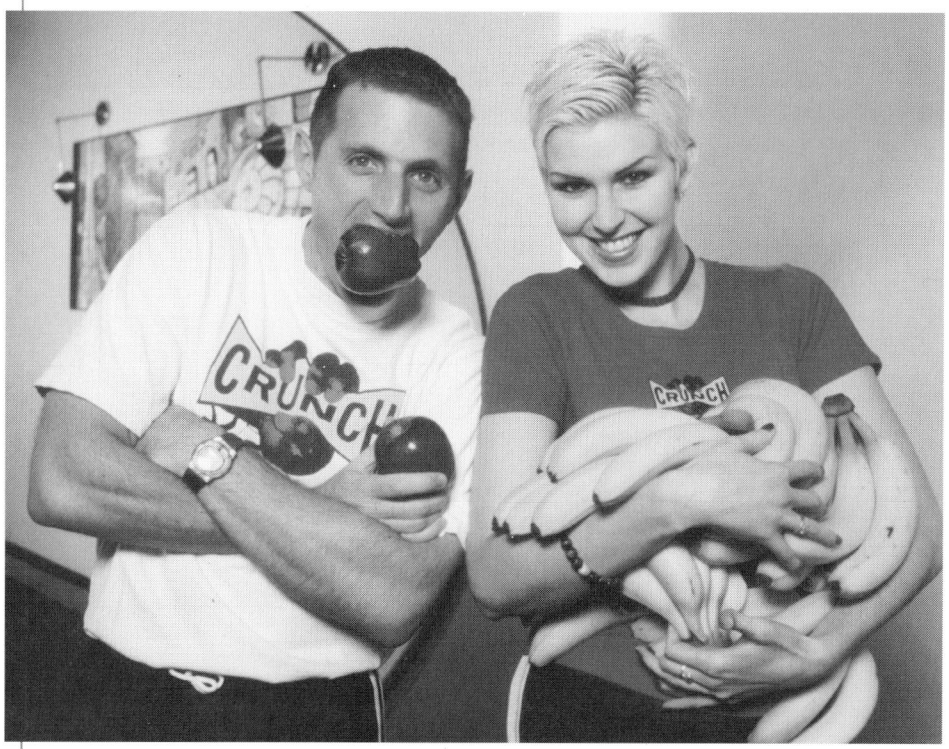

**Larry Krug** is the co-founder of the Eatwize™ Program. He has a Master's Degree in exercise physiology and served as a nutrition and training consultant for the 1996 Olympic Games. He has appeared on CNN, Dateline NBC, and E-Channel, and his nutritional and training advice has been covered in *Newsweek, Allure, Redbook, Cosmopolitan,* and *US* magazines.

**Jennifer Nardini** is both a professional journalist and personal nutritionist at CRUNCH Los Angeles. She is currently Head of Research and Development for the Eatwize™ Program and uses the method to help her own clients reach their goals. After graduating from the University of Washington with an education in both nutrition and journalism, she co-founded the Healthy Eating Rules (H.E.R.) Club, a nutritional and weight-loss support forum on the *Self Magazine* Web site. The H.E.R. Club can be accessed online at www.phys.com.

# PART I
# STEP 1: ADMITTING YOU'RE A WORKAHOLIC

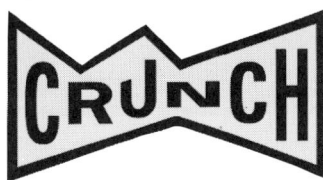

In today's fast-paced society, we always seem to have one eye on the clock. We communicate by fax, e-mail, and portable cell phones. We eat by microwave and McDonald's. We shop, bank, and invest online. We live by the adage "time is money," and we see no virtue in patience. Why?

More and more, our employers seem to judge us solely on how productive we are. The media teaches us to believe that to be successful and happy, we must be busy every minute of every day. And so work cuts into family time, socializing, romance, vacation—until we can't separate work from the rest of our lives. Work *is* our lives.

Admit it—we're all workaholics. But not all workaholics are alike. Some folks, let's call them the Movers, thrive on the frenzy. They love their work; it is their passion. People may tell them that they have Type A personalities, that they're "control freaks" who don't like to delegate authority, and that they're perfectionists with short tempers and little tolerance for mistakes. But Movers don't want to change—they don't see anything wrong with being perfectionists or loving what they do.

Other folks, let's call this group the Shakers, are whipped by the constant demands on their time. They struggle to keep up. They worry about whether they'll meet deadlines, miss opportunities, and measure up. They freely admit they feel overworked, and they welcome ways to cope.

# THE WORKAHOLIC'S WORKOUT

The Movers seem to have boundless energy. They are remarkably focused and determined. But their single-mindedness keeps them from realizing just how tired their bodies and minds really are. They tend to neglect their nutrition and ignore physical signs of deteriorating health. They are prime candidates for stress-related illnesses, such as heart disease.

The Shakers are frazzled and chronically exhausted. They may try to relax, but can't. In an attempt to soothe their nerves and ease their minds, they may overindulge in unhealthy pleasures—fatty foods, alcohol, caffeine.

No matter which kind of workaholic you are, the health consequences of overwork can be severe. You may not even realize you're tired or unfit. If you constantly feel as though you're on the run, how could you be out of shape? If you barely have time to eat meals, how could you be overweight? The workaholic's lifestyle itself promotes weight gain, high blood pressure, back pain, muscle imbalances, and a host of other problems that can lead to serious disease. And ignoring signs of poor health is easier than you think—especially when you're mind is on work.

In fact, you may not even realize how firmly workaholism has you in its grips. Take the following 20-question quiz. Give yourself one point for each question to which you answer "yes."

1. Do you consistently work more than 40 hours a week?
2. Do you routinely have to cancel plans with family and friends because you have to work late?
3. Do you usually take work to bed with you?
4. Do you frequently work on weekends?
5. Do you take work with you on vacation?
6. Do you work or read during meals?
7. Do you do work during your commute to and from the office?
8. Do you get frustrated with co-workers who are not as dedicated to their jobs as you are, or who have priorities outside the office?
9. Do you have trouble delegating authority? Do you prefer to do extra work yourself because you think that others won't be able to do it as well—or that others won't do it at all?
10. Is your datebook completely filled in for more than one week ahead?
11. Do you fear losing your job if you don't work long hours?
12. Do you constantly worry about your financial future?
13. Is work the last thing you think about before you fall asleep at night?

## STEP 1: ADMITTING YOU'RE A WORKAHOLIC

### TIPS FOR REHAB

- Take a short break from work every two hours.
- Learn to delegate tasks to co-workers, family, and friends. Don't be ashamed to ask for help.
- Focus on eating meals slowly. Try to eat meals with other people.
- Take a yoga class and learn about meditation.
- Think about the arts and crafts, sports, or hobbies you enjoyed as a child. Take one up as a hobby now.
- Turn off the television before you go to bed.
- Make time for exploring your religious or spiritual beliefs.
- Once a week, make a list of non-work-related things you want to do for yourself that week.
- Do volunteer work once a week.

14. Do you talk about work more than any other subject?
15. Do you have any non-work-related hobbies?
16. Is your idea of relaxation taking the phone off the hook while working?
17. Do you prefer to take your vacation time one or two days at a time, rather than in week-long or two-week-long stretches?
18. Do you wake up tired in the morning?
19. Do you consistently feel harried?
20. Do you often find yourself trying to do two things at once?

### SCORING

**1-5 points:** You may be in the beginning stages of workaholism, but you haven't lost control. Your work patterns tend to ebb and flow in healthy cycles.

**6-15 points:** You're a workaholic, all right, but not necessarily a willing one. With a little determination, you can easily incorporate healthy habits into your busy lifestyle.

**16-20 points:** You may think you're in control, but workaholism has gotten the best of you. You probably deny

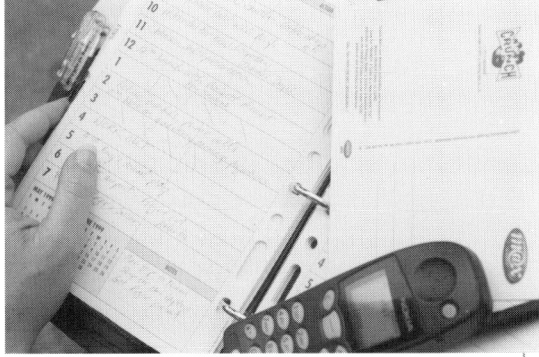

that your behavior could be affecting your long-term health. But consider this: a little time spent on yourself can translate into greater work productivity.

## THE HEALTHY WORKAHOLIC

You may have no desire to slow down or decrease your workload. Or, you may dream about taking a break, but realistically know that it'll take winning the lottery before you're able to do so. So if you must be a workaholic, how can you be a healthier, more productive one?

First of all, you need to exercise. If your job consists mainly of sitting at a desk all day, you need to work your body the way you work your mind. But that doesn't mean you'll need to take a time-management seminar to incorporate a workout into your busy schedule. Even brief, 30-minute workouts can deliver long-lasting health benefits. And we're not just talking about losing weight. After a workout:

- You'll have more energy during the day
- You'll sleep better at night
- You'll feel mentally refreshed

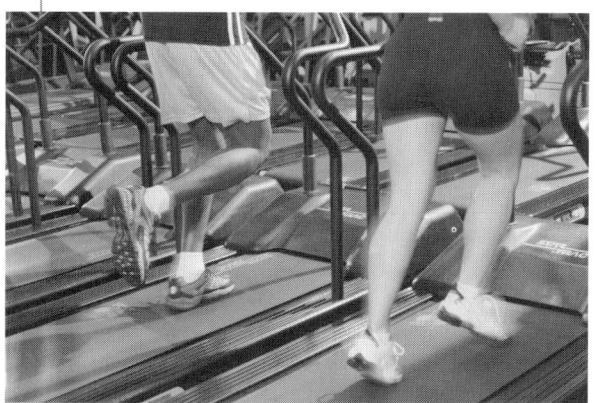

Another benefit of exercise is stress reduction. In fact, exercise is the simplest and most effective means of reducing stress. It can lower blood pressure, increase vigor, and, according to an article in *USA Today*, promote clear thinking—thereby increasing work productivity, performance, and the ability to make complex decisions by 70% ("The Physician and Sports Medicine," May 12, 1992). Exercise also releases endorphins, hormones that produce a sense of happiness and well-being.

Diet is another important component of health. If you are like most workaholics, you eat a fast-food lunch at your desk, snack on foods with high-sugar content, and drink lots of coffee, soda, or other caffeinated beverages. These unhealthy eating habits can wreak havoc with your system, depleting nutrients, adding fat, and depriving you of restful sleep.

## STEP 1: ADMITTING YOU'RE A WORKAHOLIC

If you can't imagine getting through the day without plenty of sugar and caffeine, consider this: a healthy diet can give you sustained energy, keep you just as alert, and help you avoid sudden cravings, after-lunch "lows," and sugar "crashes." Here's how:

- Eat breakfast every day—and not just any breakfast. Choose whole-grain cereals and breads and always have some form of protein—eggs, yogurt, low-fat cream cheese—which is a slow-burning energy source that will keep you mentally alert until lunch.
- Make sure you drink water throughout the day, especially if you're a coffee drinker. Coffee can dehydrate you, as can the dry air in most offices. Water helps keep you alert and refreshed.
- Eat lunch slowly. Pack a healthy lunch to work rather than eating fast food. Don't eat too much or load up on meat or other protein-rich food—it can make you sluggish in the afternoon.
- Bring fruit to snack on in the afternoon so you won't be tempted to raid the candy machine.
- As an alternative to coffee, choose a drink that contains ginseng or kava kava, herbal energy boosters that do not have the negative effects of caffeine.
- If you need help falling asleep at night, don't drink alcohol or take sleeping pills. Also, avoid eating a heavy meal within two hours of going to bed. Instead, drink chamomile or valerian root tea, which can help relax you. Also, foods high in tryptophan, an amino acid, promote sleep, so eating one of the following foods before bedtime may help you drift off more easily: turkey, bananas, figs, dates, yogurt, tuna, whole grain crackers, or nut butter. At bedtime, try to avoid alcohol, caffeine, sugar, tobacco, cheese, chocolate, sauerkraut, bacon, ham, sausage, eggplant, potatoes, spinach, and tomatoes. These foods contain tyramine, which increases the release of norepinephrine, a brain chemical stimulant.

For a more complete nutritional program that will provide you with all the energy you need for a hectic day—*and* help you lose weight, see Part 4, Eating Well.

Often, the hardest thing for a workaholic to do is to schedule time just for himself or herself. But if you can squeeze an extra 30 minutes a day into your schedule for a workout, you'll see just how beneficial time spent on yourself can be. Eventually, you may even be able to schedule a whole vacation to yourself—and you'll be in good shape to enjoy it!

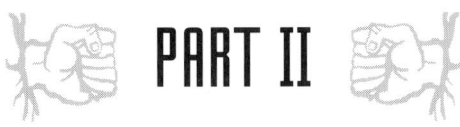

# PART II
# STEP 2: WORKING IN THE WORKOUT

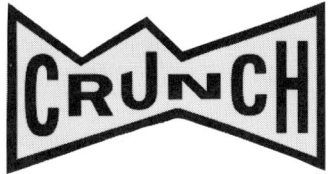

The goal of every workaholic is to get his or her work done as quickly and efficiently as possible. Why spend two hours drawing graphs for a sales report when your computer can create the graphs in 10 minutes? Why spend an hour and a half in the gym when you can get the same benefits and results from a 30-minute workout?

The truth is, you can run on a treadmill all day, every day and it's not going give you the same fitness benefits as a well-rounded workout that takes only 30 minutes, six days a week. It's the quality of the exercise you do that counts—not necessarily the quantity.

Having a well-rounded workout is key. Every good exercise program contains three main components: cardiovascular training, strength training, and flexibility training. You should do strength training only three days a week. That's because as you work each muscle, you create little tears or "traumas" in them. It is when the muscle repairs those little traumas that it becomes stronger and more toned. But your body can do this repair work only when you're resting. If you work out the same muscle two days in a row, those little traumas may turn into major traumas—i.e., injuries!

You should, therefore, alternate your strength training days with cardio training days. And always take one day a week off and *rest*. (More on how to do that in Chapter 3.)

## THE WORKAHOLIC'S WORKOUT

# FLEXIBLE MUSCLES ON A TIGHT SCHEDULE

Of the three components, flexibility training is something you can and should do before every workout. Flexibility training is simply stretching. Before you stretch, though, you should always warm up with some light cardio activity, such as jogging or jumping rope for 5 or 10 minutes. Doing so releases synovial fluid, a lubricant for your joints and ligaments that helps prevent pulls and tears.

Here are 8 basic stretches to do before every workout. Try to hold each stretch for about 15 seconds. Your stretching routine should take you less than 5 minutes.

# WORK OUT WHILE YOU WORK

When you're sweatin' on the treadmill or Stairmaster, you've probably tried to prop a newspaper on the controls and catch up on the news. Or, if your gym has televisions mounted on the walls, you may have tuned in to CNN. But what if you could get on a stationary bike, log onto the Net, and check stock quotes, do some research, or shop?

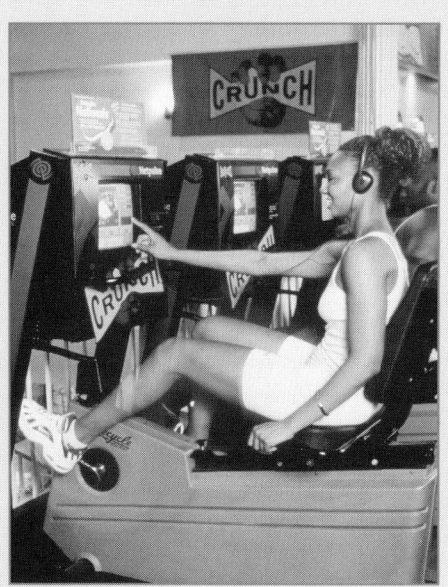

That's right. CRUNCH understands how its workaholic members feel and has introduced Netpulse Stations in its gyms. Each minute spent training on Netpulse equipment earns exercisers frequent flyer miles, free compact disks from Tower Records and Blockbuster Music, gift certificates to selected retailers, fantasy vacations, and other rewards. Netpulse Stations are ideal for busy professionals who barely have time to get to the gym—the technology allows exercisers to surf the Web, read an online newspaper or magazine, check sports scores, receive stock quotes and place trades, watch TV, listen to CDs, or even shop!

## STEP 2: WORKING IN THE WORKOUT

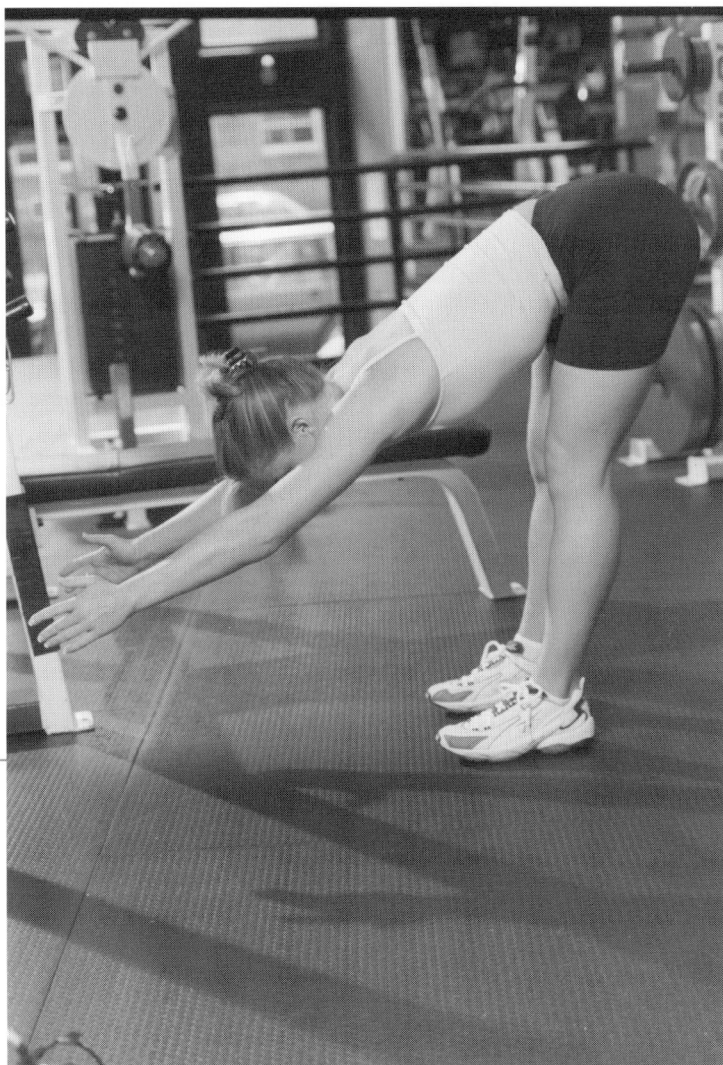

**Hamstring stretch**

Stand with your feet slightly apart. Bend your torso down to a 45 degree angle to your hips. Keep your back flat and stretch your arms out in front of you.

# THE WORKAHOLIC'S WORKOUT

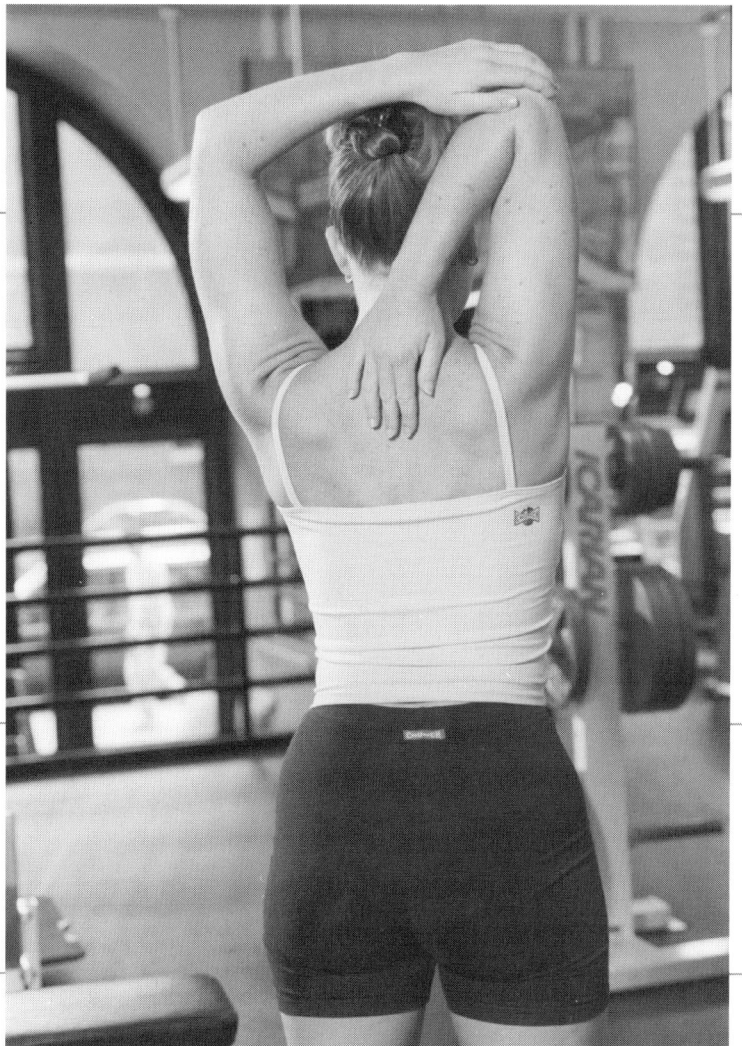

### Tricep stretch

While standing, raise one arm straight up over your head. Bend it at the elbow so that your hand falls behind your head. With the opposite arm, reach in back of you and grasp your elbow. Gently pull down on the raised arm. Switch arms.

# STEP 2: WORKING IN THE WORKOUT

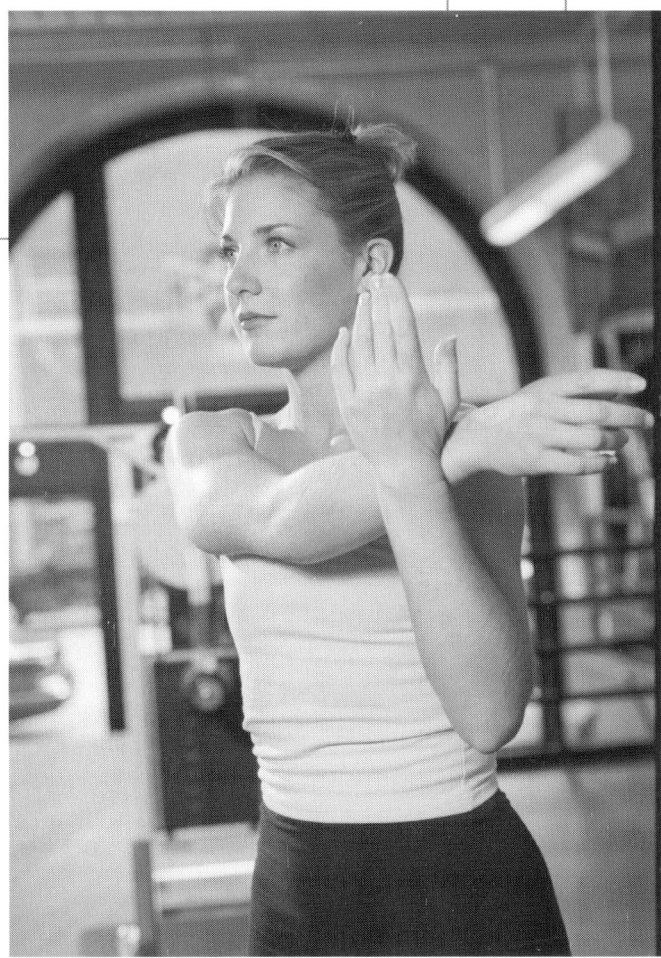

## Shoulder stretch

Place your right arm on a diagonal across your chest. With your left arm, gently pull your right arm closer into your body. Repeat on the opposite side.

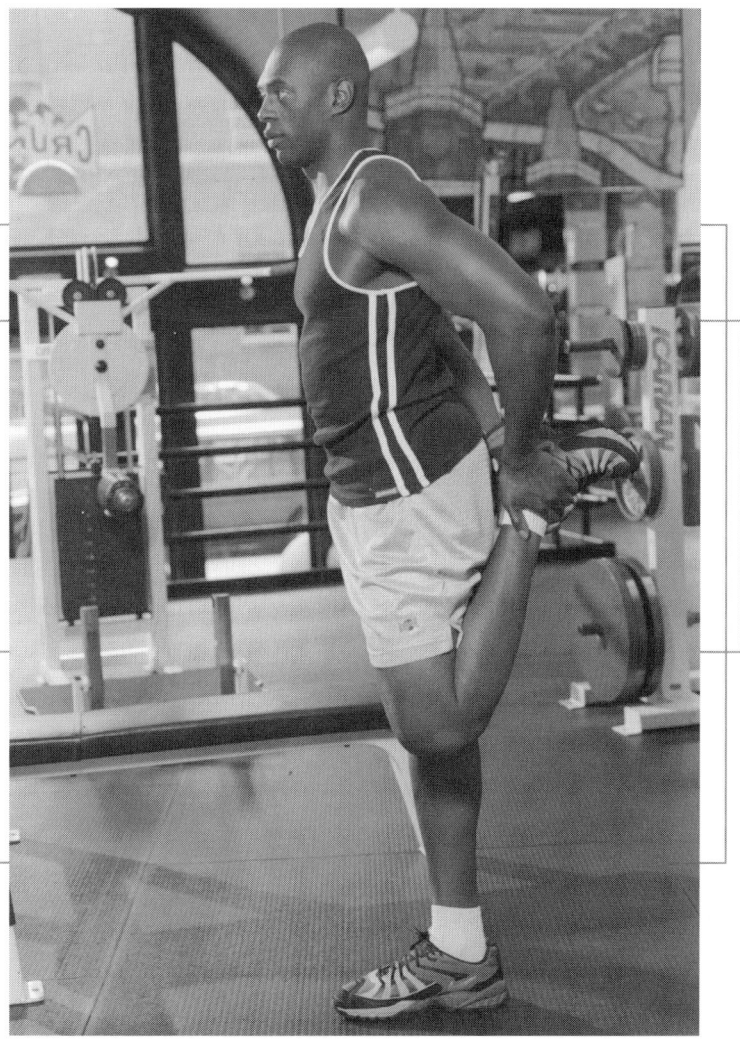

### Quad stretch

Stand straight with your feet together. Bend one knee and with both hands grab onto your ankle. Gently pull the ankle up toward your butt. Keep your thighs and knees parallel and your back straight. Do not swing your bent knee out to the side. Repeat with the opposite side.

## STEP 2: WORKING IN THE WORKOUT

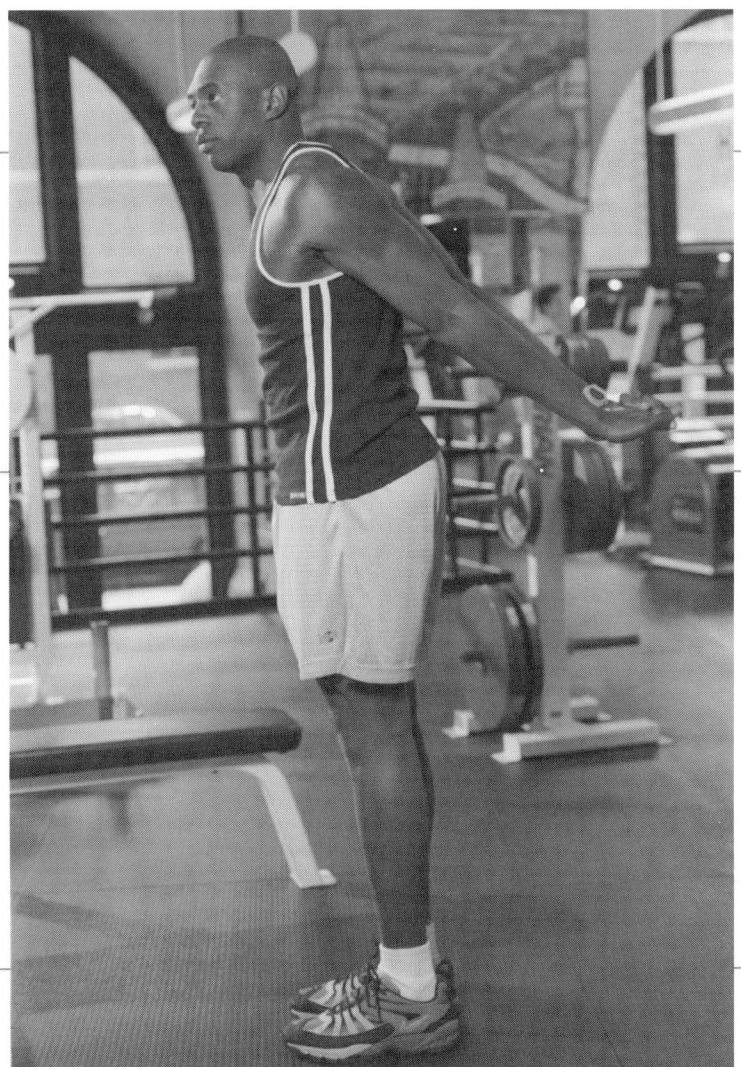

**Chest stretch**

Clasp hands together behind your back and thrust your chest out.

# THE WORKAHOLIC'S WORKOUT

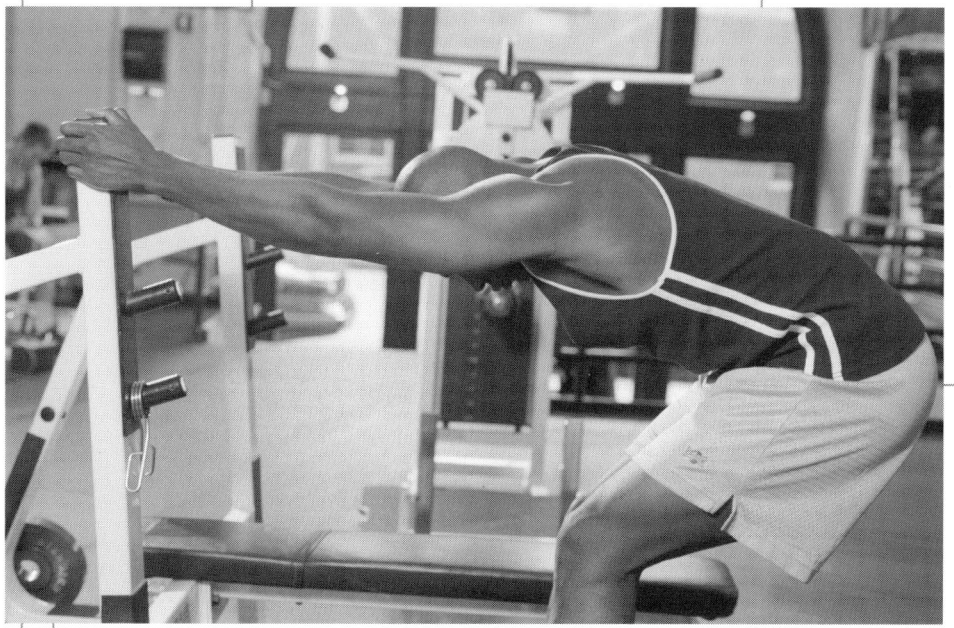

**Back stretch**

With your feet together, stand about a foot away from a stable pole. Grab onto the pole at at about shoulder height. Lean back, sitting slightly. Keep your head down.

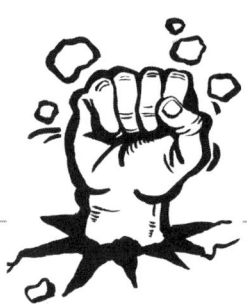

## STEP 2: WORKING IN THE WORKOUT

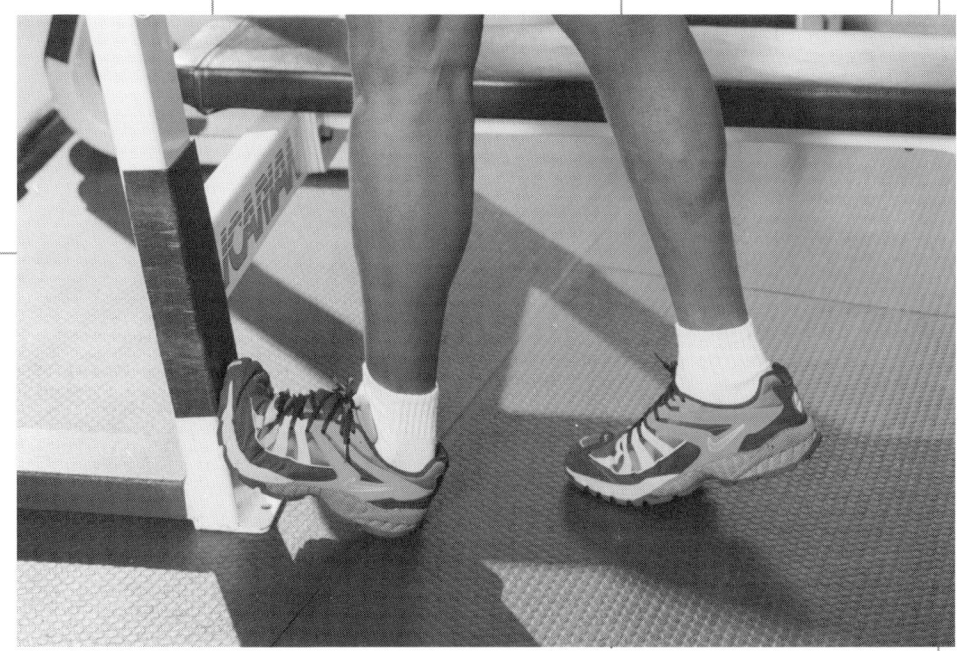

### Calf stretch

Keeping your heels firmly planted on the floor, put your toes up on a wall or pole so that you feel the stretch in your calves. Lean forward toward the wall or pole.

# THE WORKAHOLIC'S WORKOUT

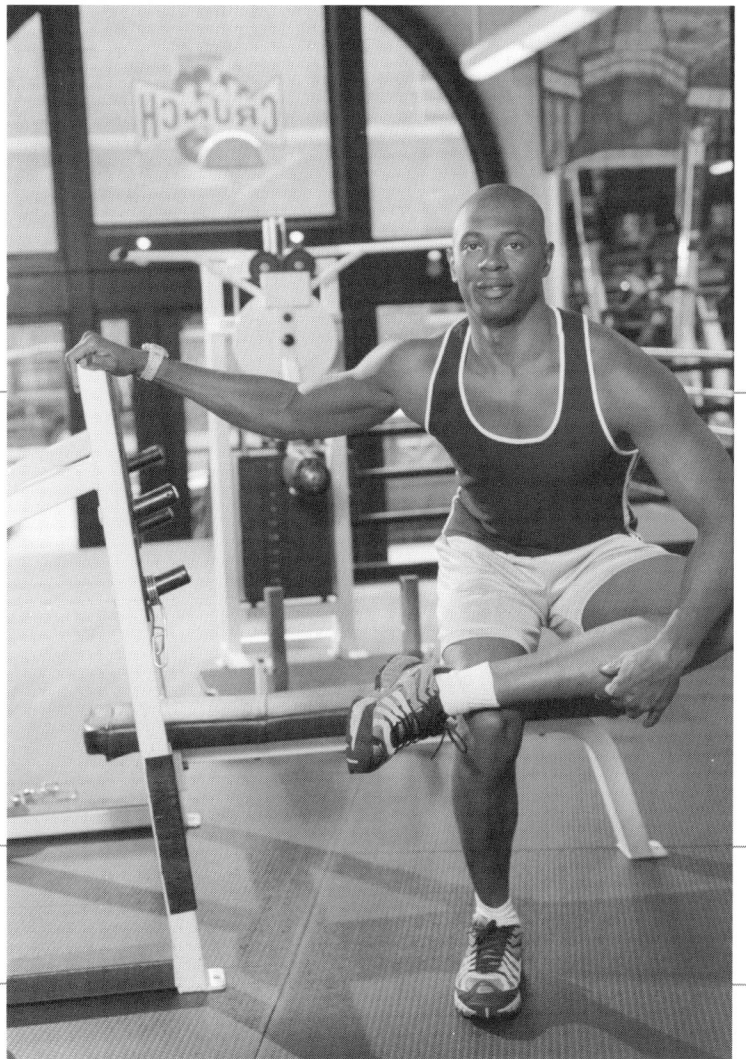

### Glute stretch

While standing and holding a stationary object for balance, cross one ankle over the opposite knee, as shown. Lower your butt toward the ground, as if you were going to sit. Keep your back straight. Repeat with the opposite side.

## STEP 2: WORKING IN THE WORKOUT

# PUT YOUR HEART INTO IT

The next workout component, cardiovascular training, targets your most important muscle—your heart. Any sport or exercise that gets your heart rate up consistently over a period of time helps to improve your heart's efficiency. Cardio training is also called aerobic exercise—the term "aerobic" refers to the amount of oxygen that's being delivered to your muscles. As your heart efficiently pumps freshly oxygenated blood to your various muscles, you're increasing your "aerobic capacity." You know when your cardiovascular fitness is improving when it takes you longer and longer to get winded when you exercise.

The goal of cardio training is to sustain activity at your target heart rate, which is 60 to 75% of your maximum heart rate. Your maximum heart rate is determined by subtracting your age from 220. Let's use a 20-year old as an example:

220 - 20 years = 200 beats per minute (bpm)
200 bpm = maximum heart rate
60 to 75% intensity = 120 to 150 beats per minute

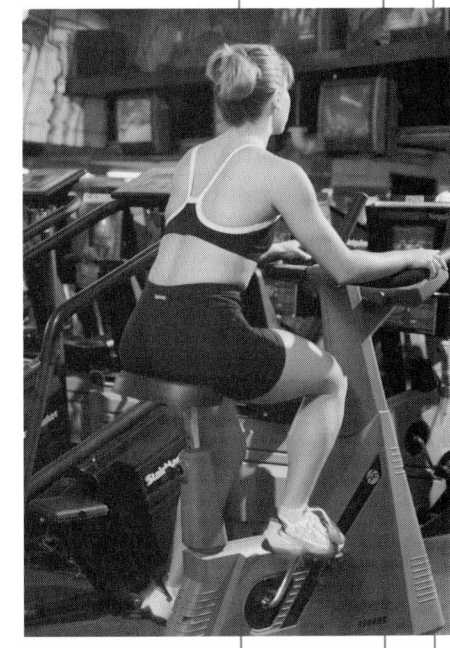

Heart rate monitors offer the most convenient readings, but a more practical approach is a six-second pulse count. Count the number of beats you feel in six seconds and multiply that by 10. For example, if our 20-year old counts 14 beats in six seconds, she is exercising at 140 beats per minute—well within her target heart rate zone.

Regular cardio workouts at your target heart rate will lower your heart rate when you're at rest. That is a good thing because it means your heart does not have to work as hard to maintain circulation when you're not exercising (which is most of the time). Your heart becomes more efficient.

You have lots of options for cardio training—walking, jogging, biking, hiking, jumping rope, doing jumping jacks, etc. Your goal should be to exercise aerobically for 20 minutes at your target heart rate.

# THE WORKAHOLIC'S WORKOUT

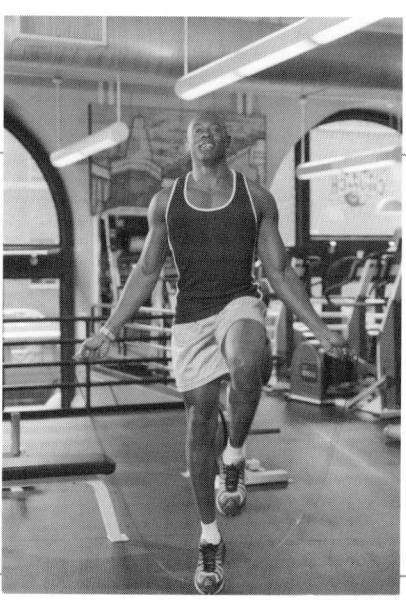
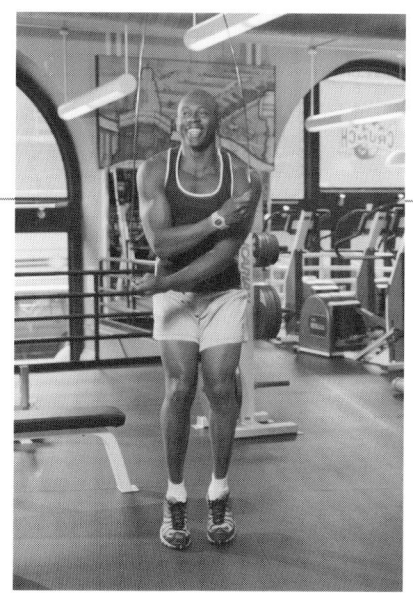

## THE CARDIO WORKOUT

You need one of the following:

- Stationary bike
- Jump rope
- Treadmill
- Stairmaster

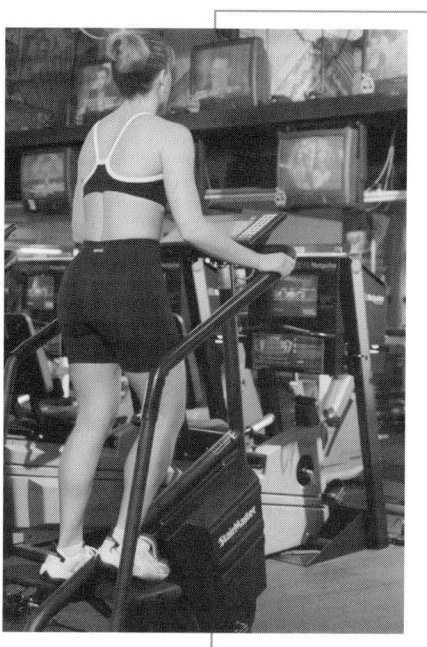

On days when you are doing only cardio training, try to exercise at your target heart rate for 20 minutes. To get the most out of the workout time, start and end the workout with five minutes of interval training. Instead of exercising at a consistent pace for the five minutes, alternate intervals of exercising at a moderate pace with intervals of exercising at a fast pace. Here is an example:

## STEP 2: WORKING IN THE WORKOUT

| minutes:seconds | exercise |
|---|---|
| 3:15 | light to moderate peddling, jumping, or jogging at a nice easy pace |
| :15 | sprint |
| :30 | slow down |
| :15 | sprint |
| :30 | slow down |
| :15 | sprint |
| **Total time:** | **5 minutes** |

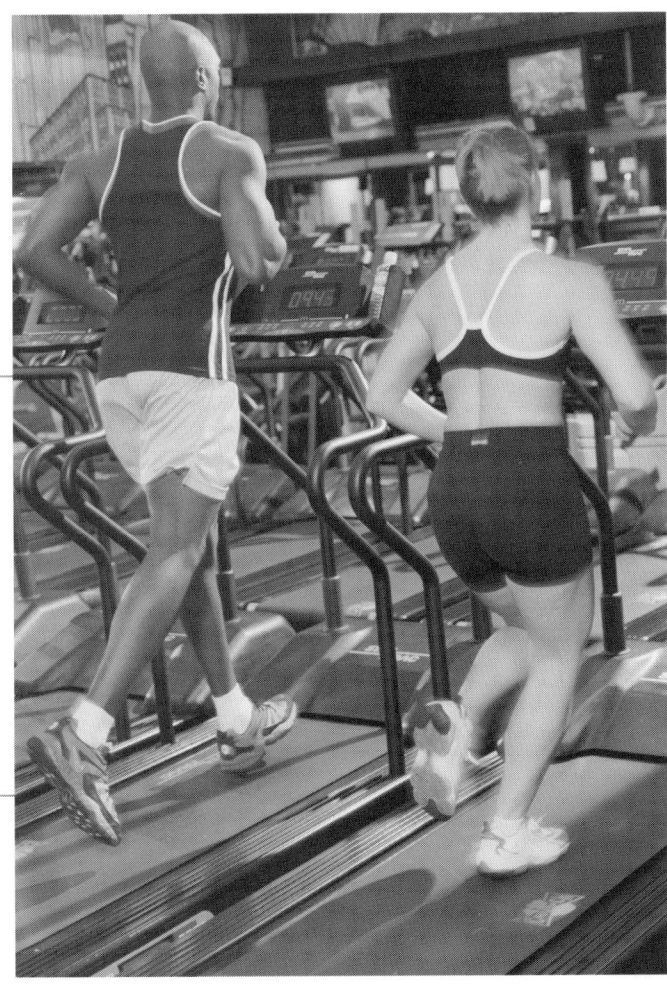

# THE WORKAHOLIC'S WORKOUT

## FULL-STRENGTH EXERCISE

On strength training days, you can choose among three strength training workouts designed to suit your schedule, no matter where you are: The Home or Office Workout, The Gym Workout, and The Business Travel Workout.

These strength training workouts are timed so that you can finish them in a half an hour. Keep your eye on the timer—by keeping your pace up, you are also giving yourself a cardiovascular workout as well as a strength workout.

The goal of these strength training workouts is to work all of the major muscle groups. People who just focus on cardio training tend to be more prone to injuries because they have greater muscle imbalances—meaning that some muscles are very developed while others are relatively weak. A full-body workout makes sure you keep all your muscles in good working order.

Here are the three strength training workouts, which are followed by detailed descriptions of how to perform each exercise safely and efficiently.

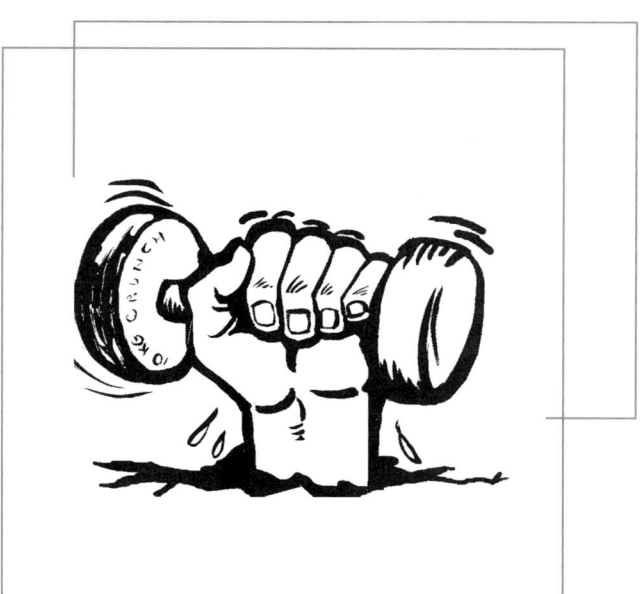

## STEP 2: WORKING IN THE WORKOUT

# THE OFFICE/HOME WORKOUT

What you need:

- Dumbbells—10 to 15 pounds
- Step with risers
- Jump rope
- Towel
- Mat
- Body bar
- Timer

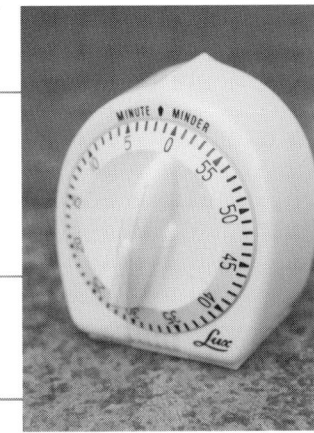

| minutes:seconds | exercise |
|---|---|
| 1:00 to 3:00 | Jump rope for about 1 to 3 minutes depending on your level of fitness |

| sets/reps | |
|---|---|
| 1 / 15 | Push-ups, from the toes, if you can, or from the knees. You are working the triceps and chest and building core stability in the abs and lower back. |
| 1 / 15 | Lunges, with a body bar onto the step |

| minutes:seconds | |
|---|---|
| 5:00 | One-legged squats—nice and slow at your own pace. |

| sets/reps | |
|---|---|
| 1 / 15 | Bicep curls with body bar |
| 1 / 15 | Bent-over rows, which work the back muscles |
| 1 / 25 | Crunches |

Repeat above routine 3 times

**Total time:**     **30 minutes**

As you get stronger and less challenged, you can add some advanced moves and challenge yourself to do more.

# THE WORKAHOLIC'S WORKOUT

## THE GYM WORKOUT

After a 10-minute cardio workout, set yourself up in the gym near the leg curl and leg extension machines.

| sets/reps | exercise |
|---|---|
| 2 / 15 | Leg curls, with weight that gives you adequate resistance |
| 2 / 15 | Leg extensions, again with weight that gives you adequate resistance |

| minutes:seconds | |
|---|---|
| :30 | Crunches |
| :15 | Break |
| :30 | Scissor kicks |
| :30 | Break |
| :30 | Leg raises |
| :30 | Push-ups |
| :30 | Shoulder presses with dumbbells or body bar |
| :15 | Break |
| :30 | Pull-downs with proper weight |
| :15 | Break |
| :30 | Bench dips |
| :15 | Break |
| :30 | Dumbbell curls |
| 2:00 | Stretch and cool down |

**Total time:**  **30 minutes**

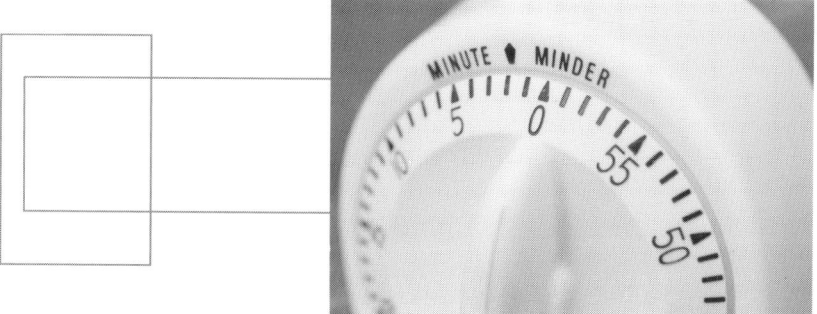

## STEP 2: WORKING IN THE WORKOUT

# THE BUSINESS TRAVEL WORKOUT

What you need:

1. Towel
2. Jump rope
3. Chair
4. Timer

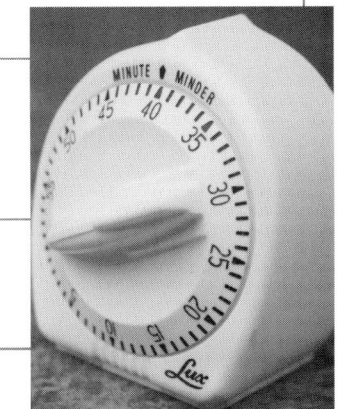

| minutes:seconds | exercise |
|---|---|
| 10:00 | Jump rope |

| sets/reps | |
|---|---|
| 3 / 15 | Push-ups |
| 3 / 15 | Crunches |
| 3 / 15 | Chair dips |
| 3 / 15 | Towel squats |

**Total time:**     **30 minutes**

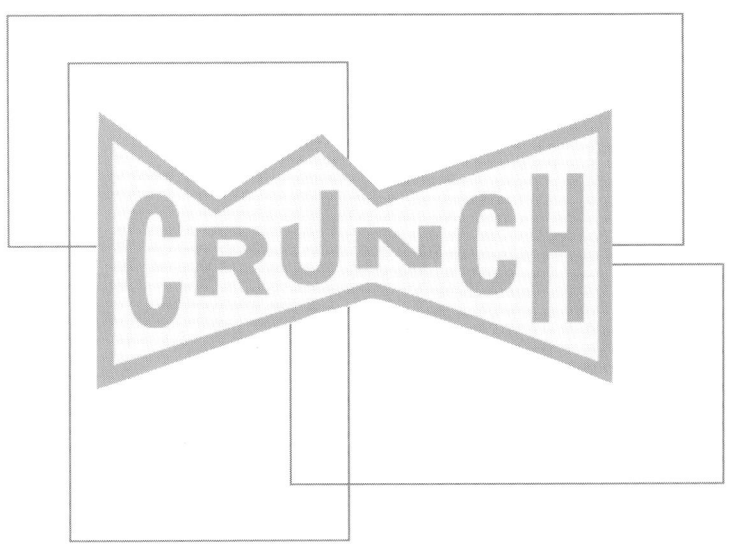

# THE WORKAHOLIC'S WORKOUT

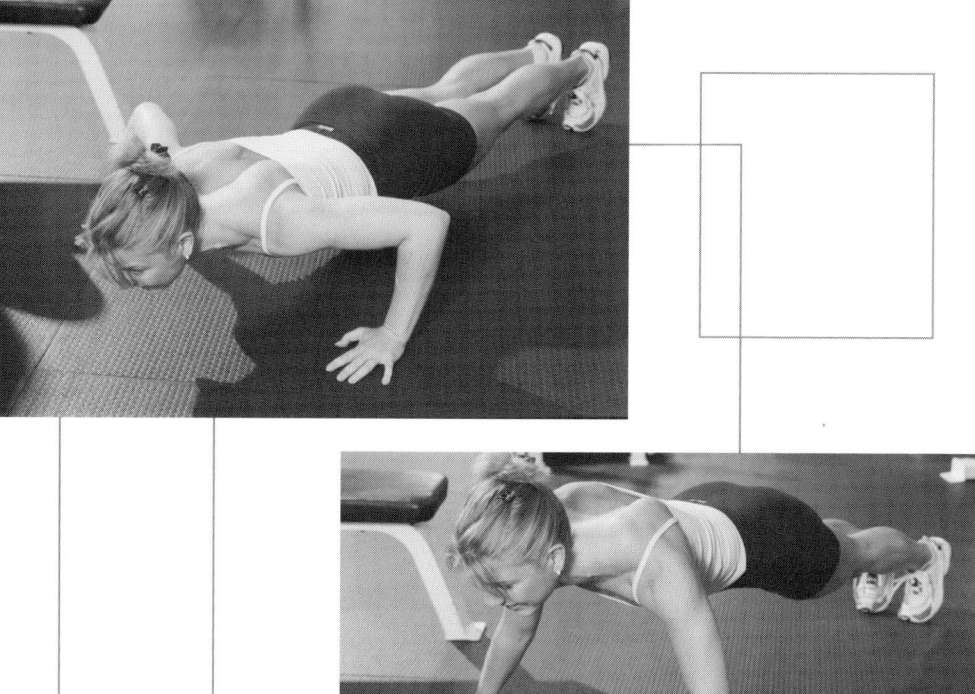

### Push-ups

You can do these from your knees, with your feet in the air, or from your toes. In either case, place your hands slightly wider than shoulder-width apart. Make sure you look forward, not down, as you do the push-ups. Keep your abs tight, your back flat (not swayed), and your head up. While push-ups mainly work the chest muscles, they also work the triceps and abs.

## STEP 2: WORKING IN THE WORKOUT

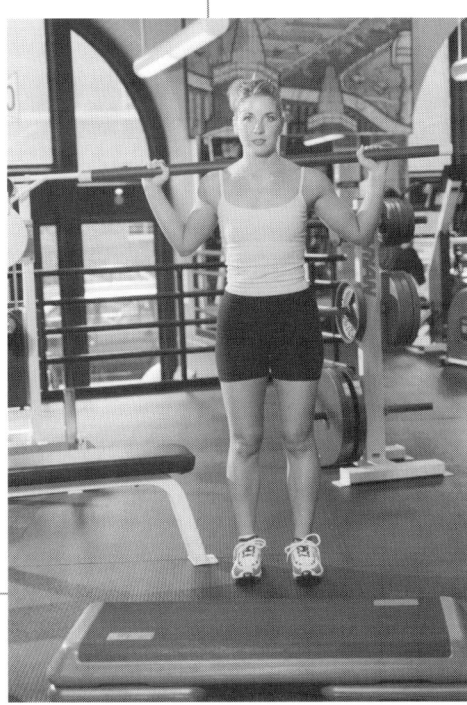

### Lunges

Place a step in front of you and hold a body bar behind your shoulders. Place one foot on the step, lunging until your opposite knee almost touches the floor. Alternate legs.

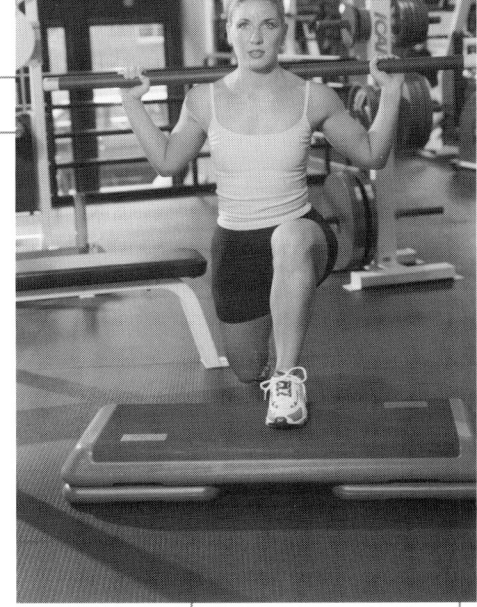

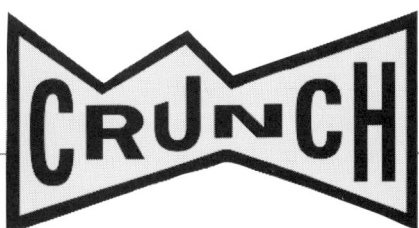

# THE WORKAHOLIC'S WORKOUT

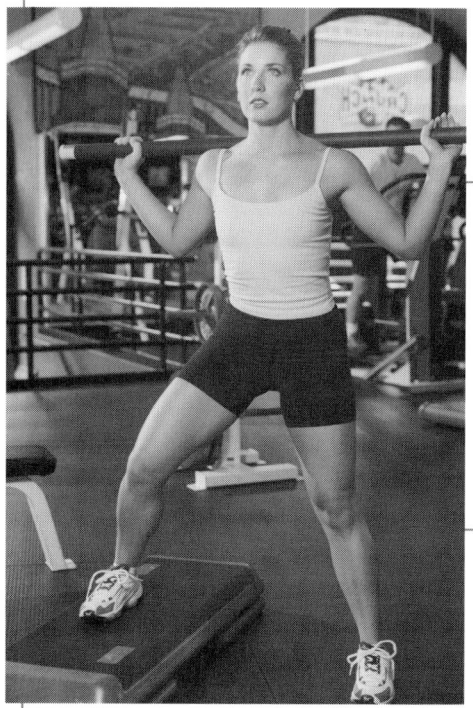

### One-legged squats

Hold a body bar across your shoulders, in back of your neck. Step to the side, onto a step, and squat. Your knees should not extend past your toes. Repeat, stepping with the opposite leg.

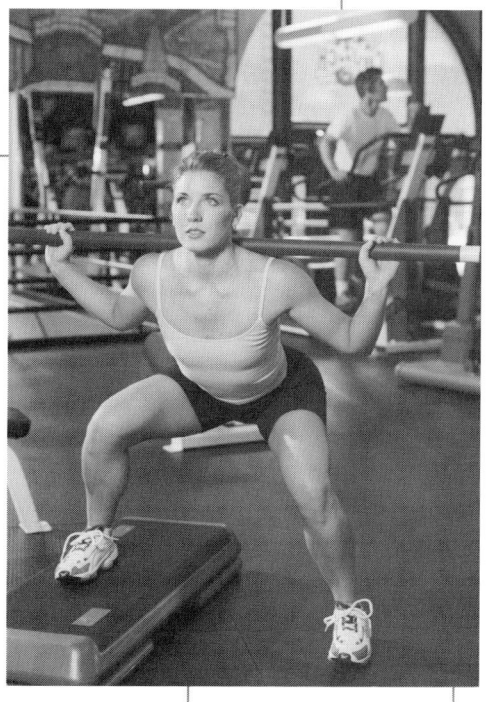

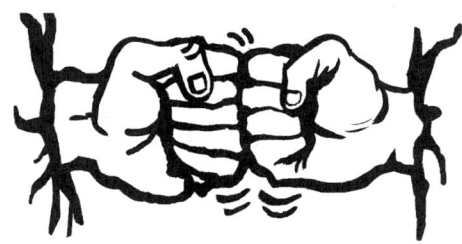

## STEP 2: WORKING IN THE WORKOUT

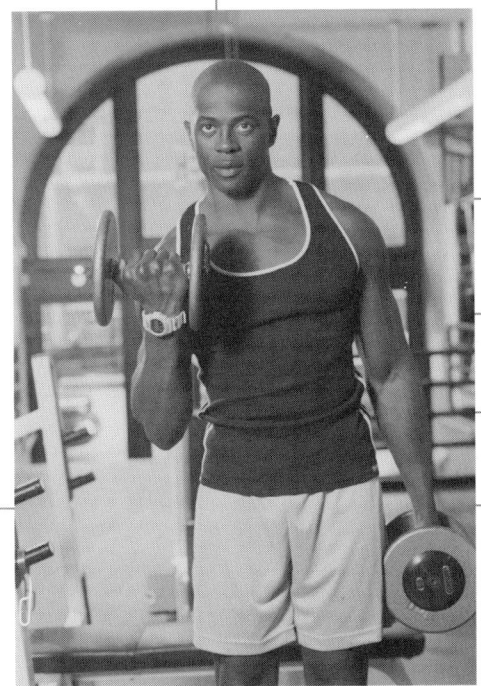 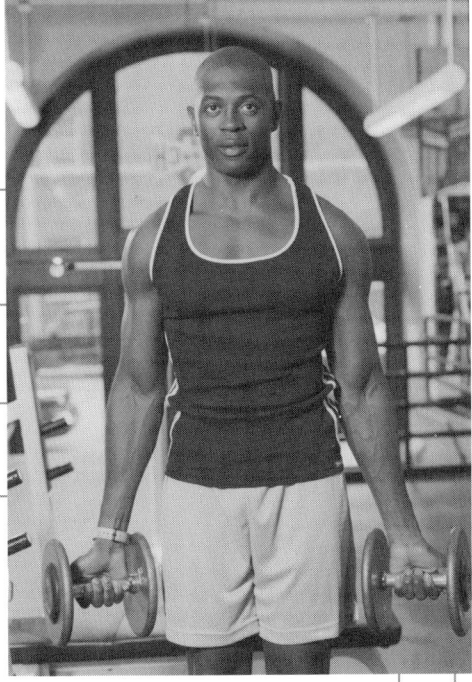

**Bicep curls with dumbbells**

Put your elbows at your sides and face your palms up. Alternating arms, lower the dumbbell toward the floor and then curl the dumbbell up to your shoulders.

# THE WORKAHOLIC'S WORKOUT

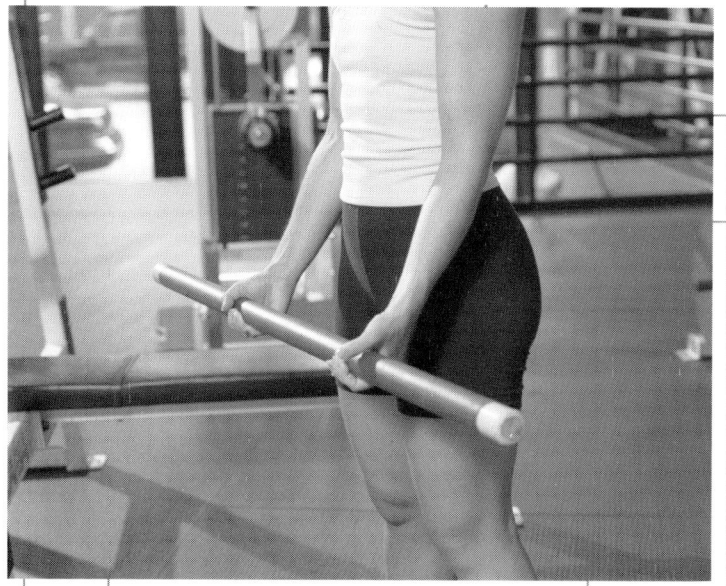

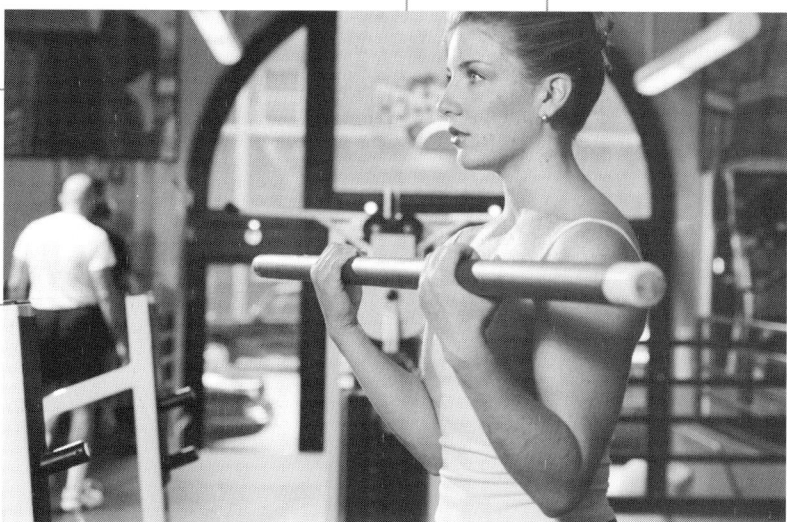

**Bicep curls with body bar**

Performing the bicep curl with a body bar instead of dumbbells works both arms simultaneously and evenly distributes the weight between them, optimizing your balance.

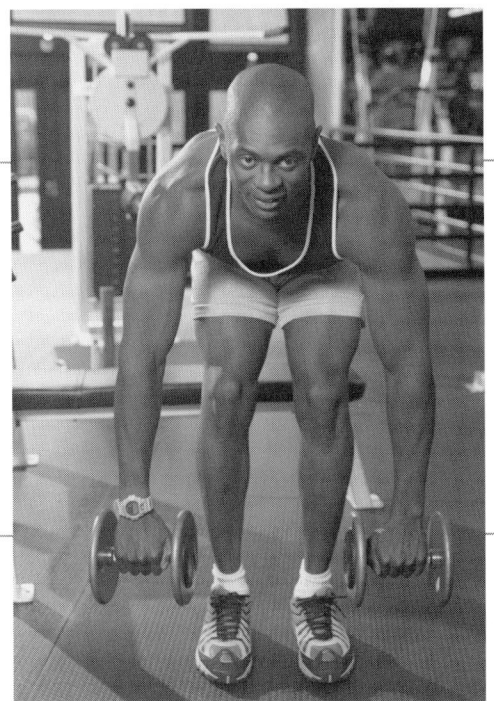

### Bent-over rows

Standing with knees soft, legs shoulder-width apart, bend from the waist to form a 45 degree angle. Your arms should be slightly bent and hands should grip the dumbbells with palms facing in, holding the weights at ankle level. Lifting from the back muscles, raise your arms to shoulder height slowly, then return to starting position.

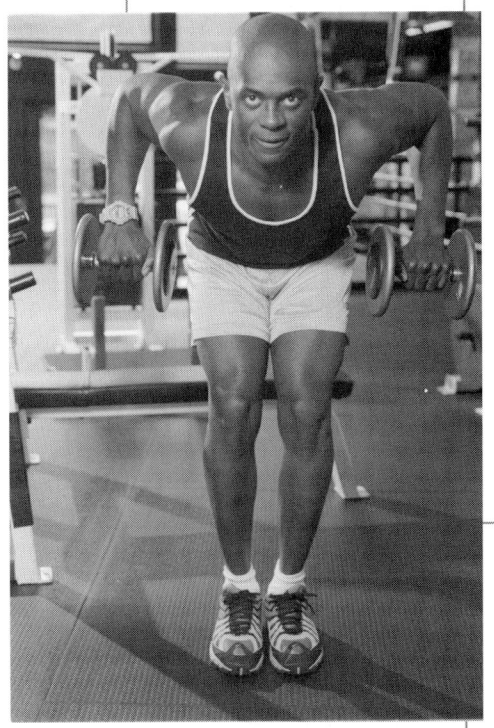

# THE WORKAHOLIC'S WORKOUT

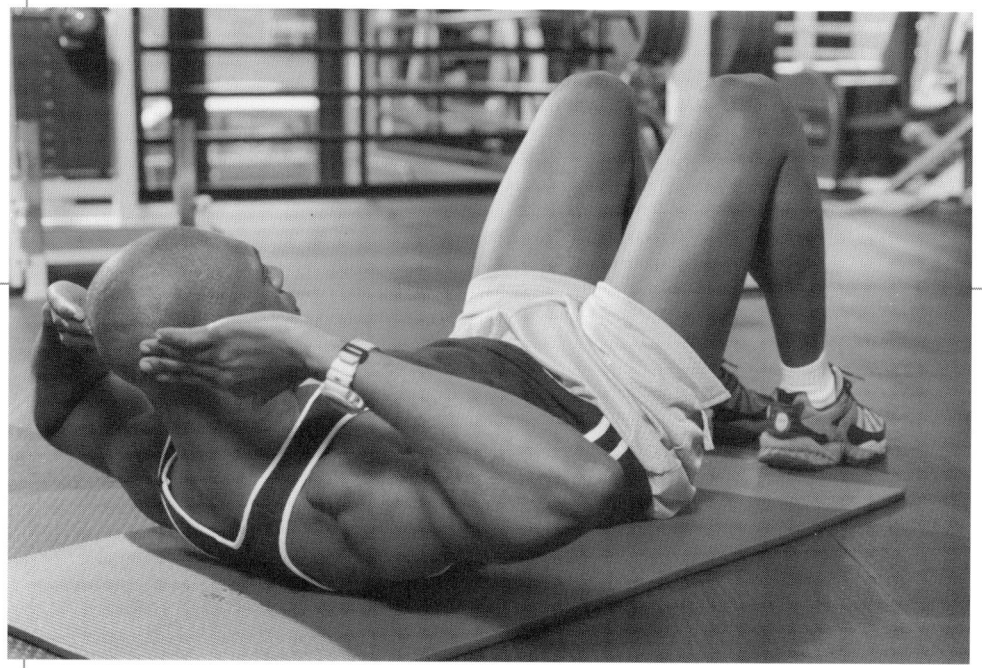

### Crunches

Lie on your back on the floor with your knees bent up and your feet flat on the floor. Place your hands behind your head, but be careful not to pull your head and neck up—your head should just be resting in your hands. Crunch up, bringing your head toward your knees and slowly lowering it again—but not all the way to the floor! Keep your shoulder blades just off the floor. Do not crane up—think of raising your rib cage.

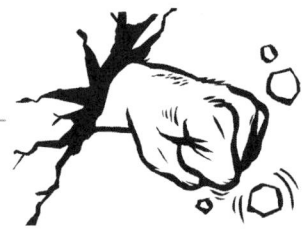

# STEP 2: WORKING IN THE WORKOUT

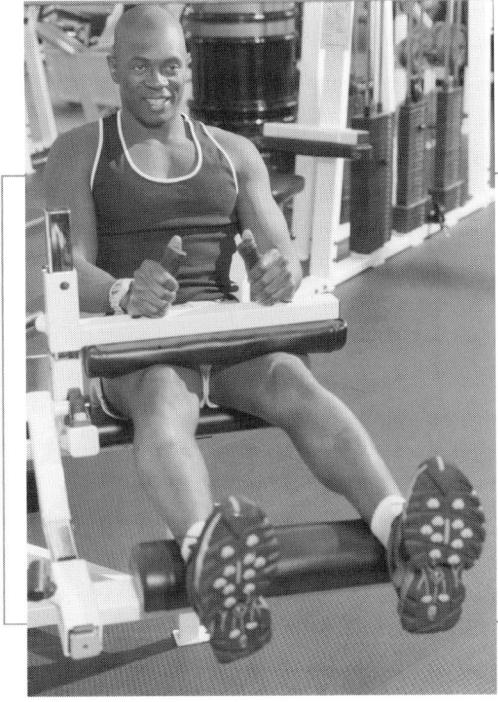

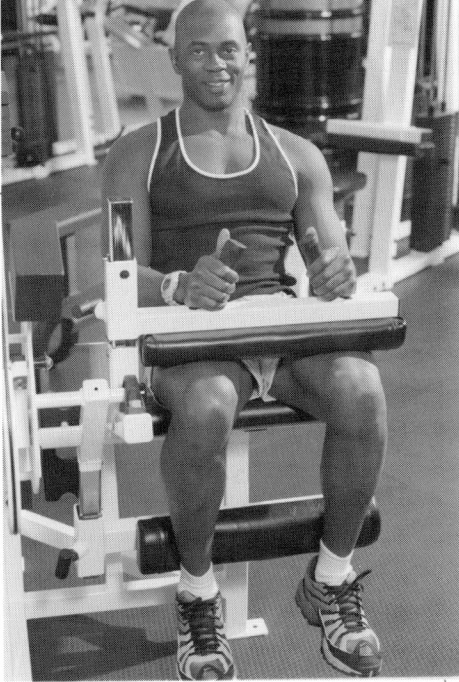

## Leg curls

Sit on the leg curl machine and hold the bars. The pad should rest on the back of your ankles. Align the axis pin to the rear of your knee by adjusting your seat back accordingly. *This is very important!* If the axis pin is not aligned correctly, you could hurt your knees. Point your toes toward the ceiling and keep your back slightly flexed so that your lower back is *not* touching the seat back. Press the pad down so that a 90 degree angle is formed between your upper and lower legs.

# THE WORKAHOLIC'S WORKOUT

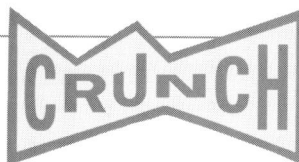

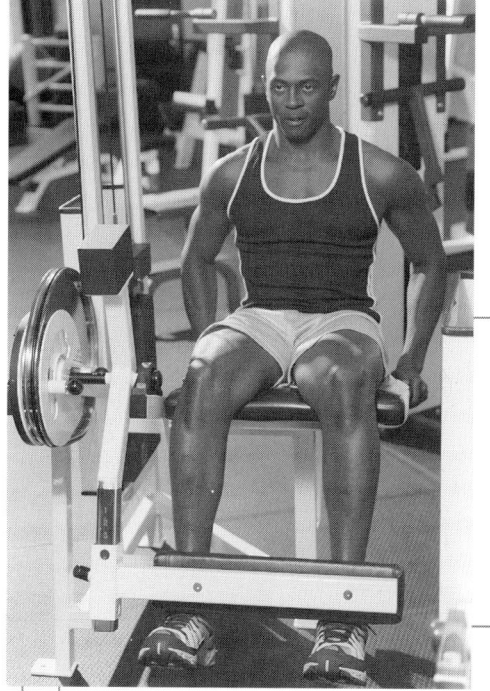

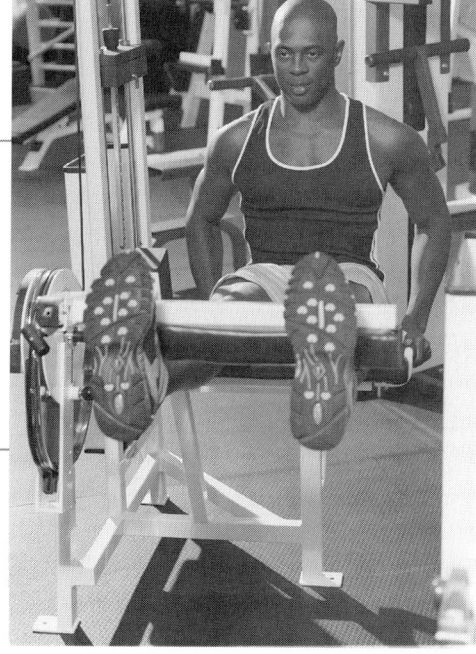

**Leg extensions**

Sit on the leg extension machine and grab the bars with both hands. Make sure the axis pin on the machine is aligned with the rear of your knee joint by adjusting the seat back accordingly. This is very important to avoid injury to your knee! The shin pad should rest just above the front ankles. Extend your legs fully, but do not lock your knee at the top. Do not bring the weight all the way down between reps.

# STEP 2: WORKING IN THE WORKOUT

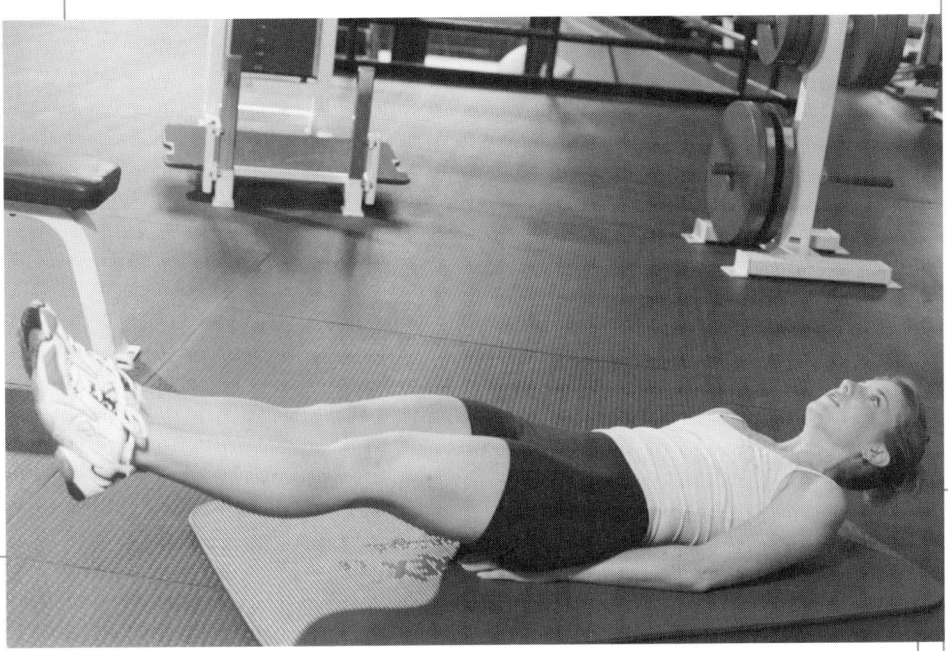

### Leg raises

Lie on your back with your arms at your sides and place your hands under your butt. Keeping your legs fully extended, raise them until they are perpendicular to your body. Lower them again, but do not lower them all the way to the floor between reps.

## THE WORKAHOLIC'S WORKOUT

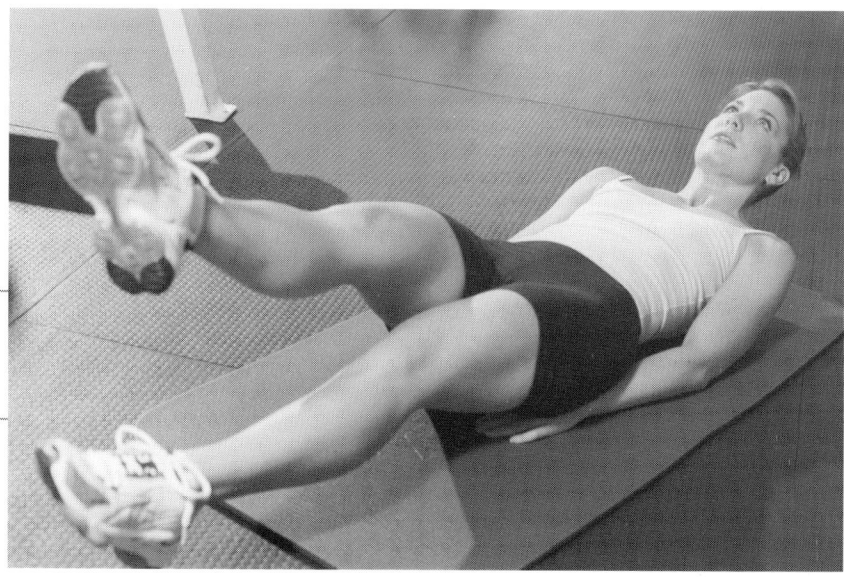

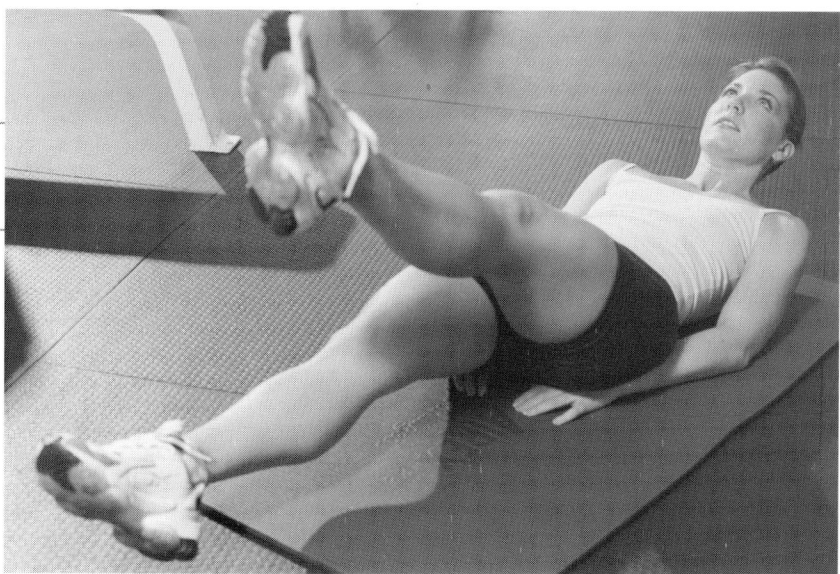

**Scissor kicks**

Lie on the floor with your arms at your sides and your hands under your buttocks. Keeping your legs fully extended, raise your legs, alternating them in a kicking motion. Bring your butt off the floor. Do not bring your legs down until the timer goes off.

## STEP 2: WORKING IN THE WORKOUT

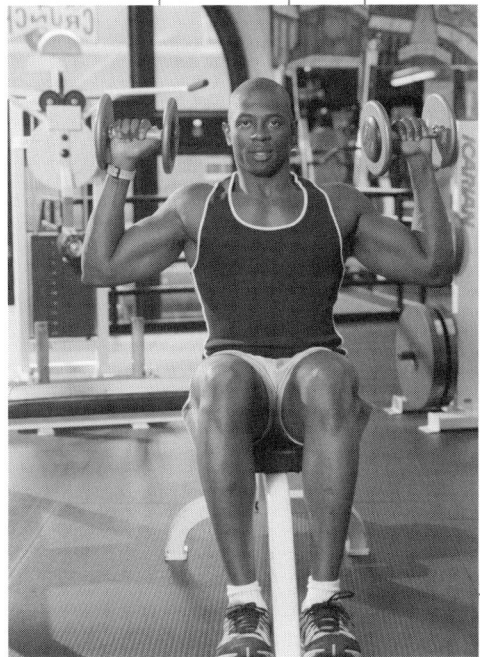

### Shoulder presses

Sit on the bench with your feet on the floor and a dumbbell in each hand. Keep your arms outstretched to your sides, and, as you lift the dumbbells over your head, bend your elbows as they reach shoulder height. This movement pushes the dumbbells toward the ceiling.

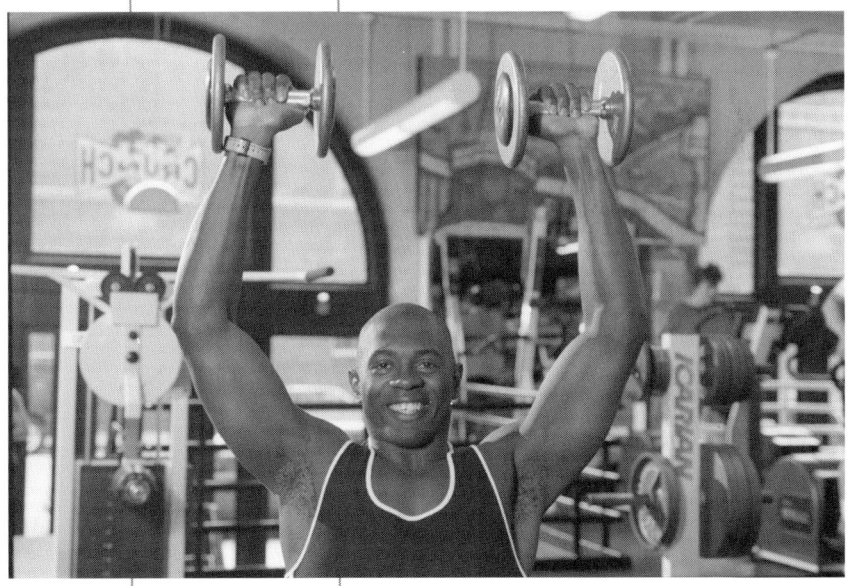

## THE WORKAHOLIC'S WORKOUT

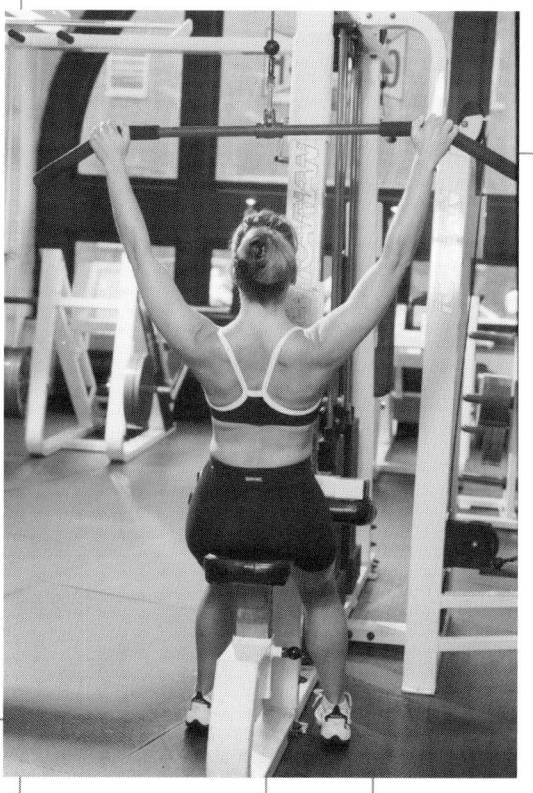

### Lat pull-downs

Sit with the pad above your thighs. With a slightly wider than shoulder-width overgrip, pull the bar to the middle of your chest. Keep your back straight. Do *not* pull down or press down behind your head—you can injure your shoulder. Unfortunately, this is a very common mistake among gym members.

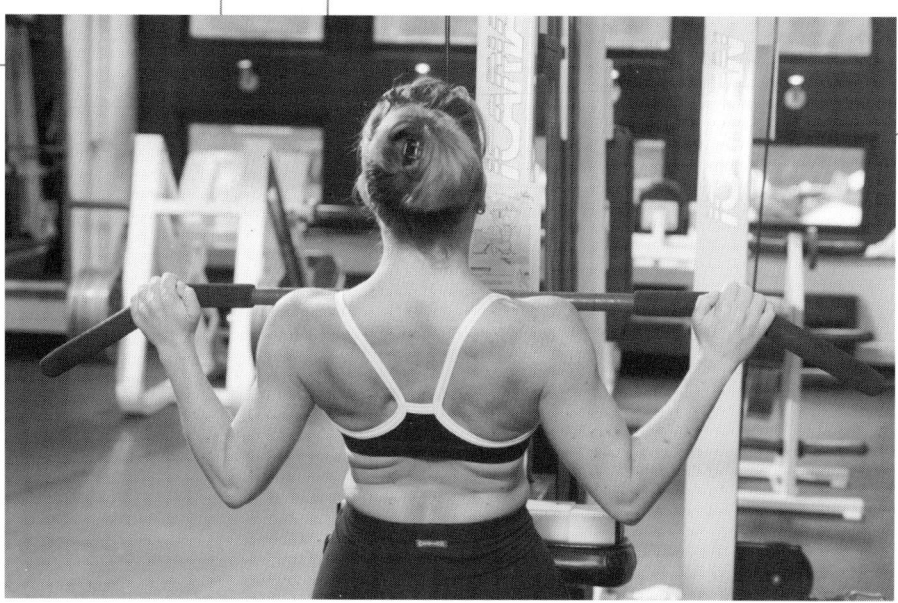

## STEP 2: WORKING IN THE WORKOUT

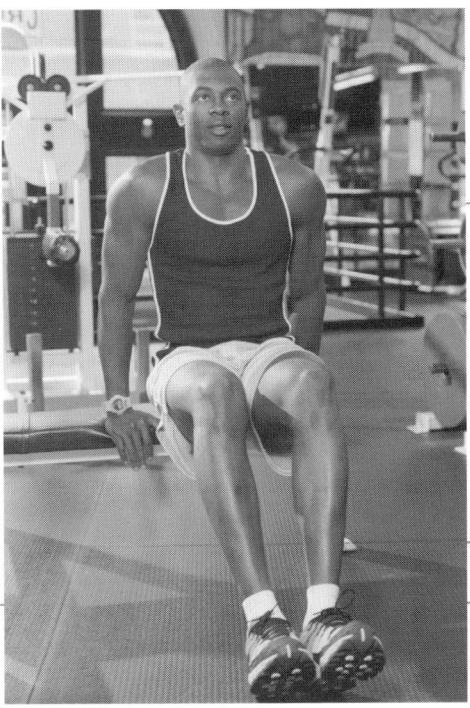

### Bench dips

Sit on the edge of a bench and grasp the edge of the bench on either side of your hips with your hands. Raise your butt up and slightly forward off the bench. Bend your knees and keep your weight on your heels, while lowering your butt toward the floor. Raise back up. Keep your back flat against the edge of the bench.

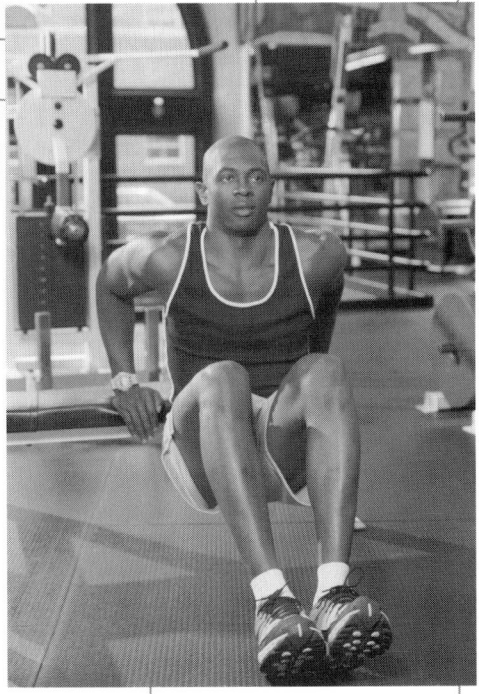

# THE WORKAHOLIC'S WORKOUT

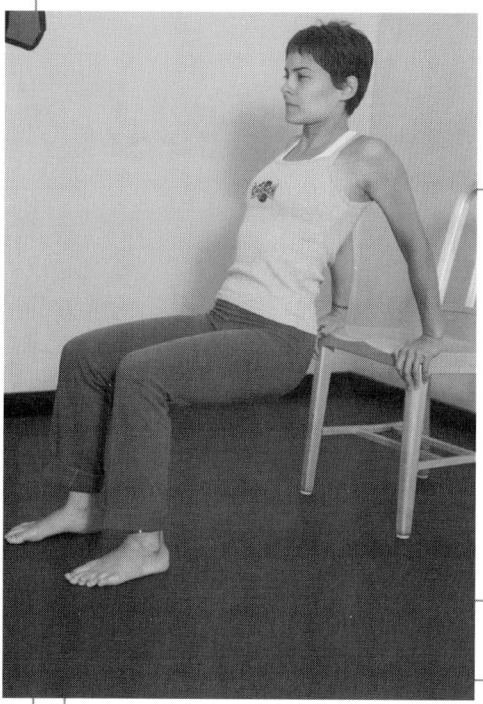

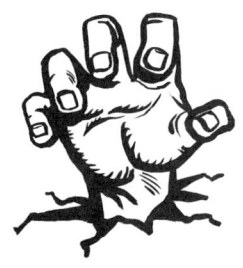

### Chair dips

You can do tricep dips using a chair instead of a bench. Make sure the chair is heavy and stable—an office swivel chair on rollers won't work!

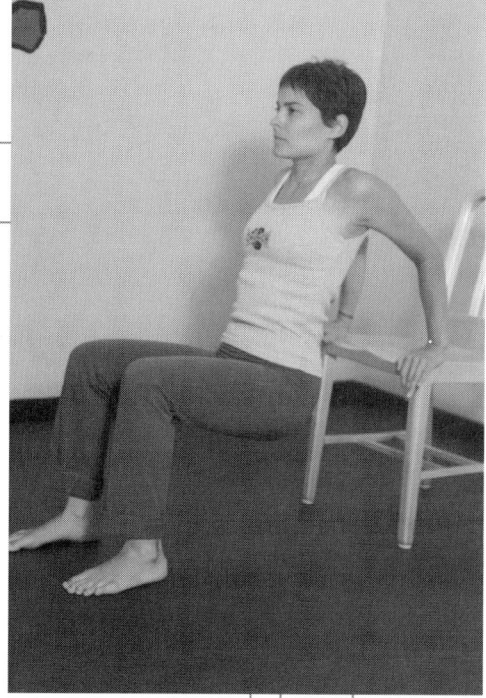

# STEP 2: WORKING IN THE WORKOUT

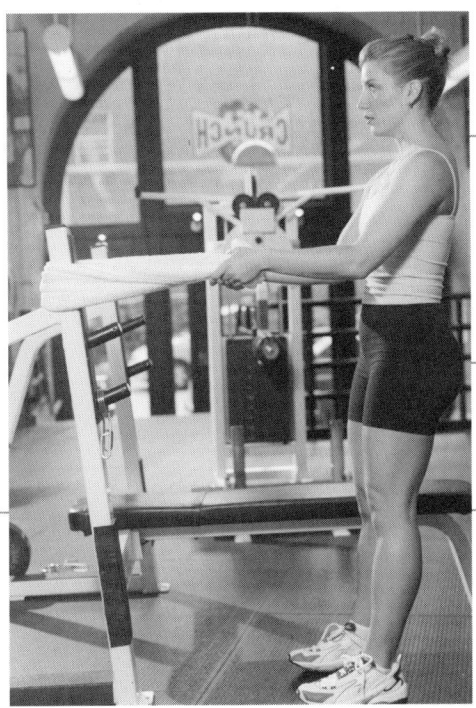

## Towel squats

These are also known as pole squats. Wrap a towel around a pole or piece of stationary equipment. Squat down while grasping the ends of the towel firmly and leaning back slightly.

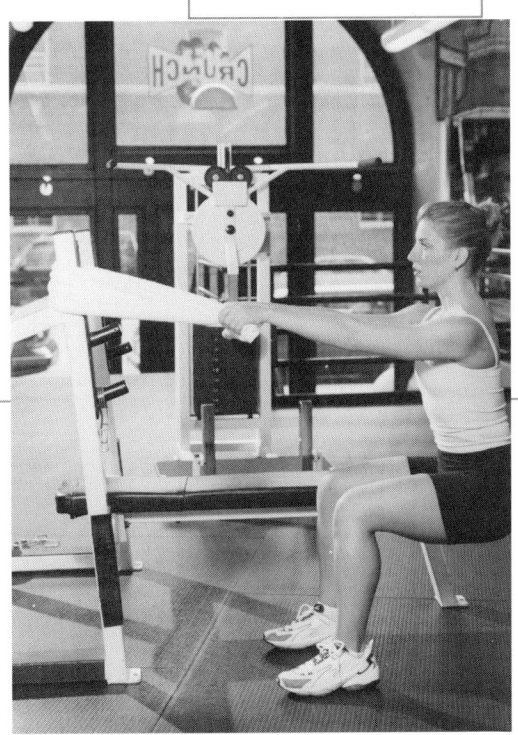

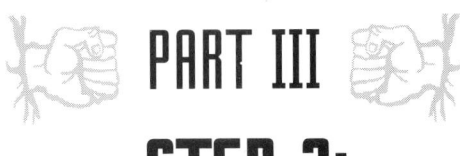

# PART III
# STEP 3:
# LEARNING HOW TO RELAX

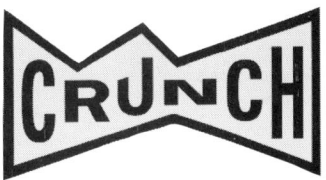

Is your idea of a vacation staying at a chain hotel with a full-service business center and an Internet hook-up in every room? Does your bathing suit have a belt you can clip your cell phone onto? Is the *Wall Street Journal* your idea of "beach reading"? Do you even remember the last time you took a vacation?

Most people can't wait for vacation. Then there's you. You have to be forced to go away for a week, don't you?

Getting you to the mountains, the beach, a spa, or a foreign city is the job of your boss, your spouse, your friends, or your doctor. Making sure your vacation destination doesn't have the word "Institute" in it, though, is our job. We're going to show you how to take "mini-vacations" during even your busiest day, so that you won't suffer complete burnout before your bags are packed.

First, relaxation really has nothing to do with sitting beneath a palm tree on a tropical island (especially if you've brought your laptop but not enough sunscreen). Relaxation has to do with learning how to release muscle tension, slow your heart rate, and clear your mind. If you can do that for just five minutes, once every couple of hours, you will actually have more energy and work more efficiently throughout the day.

# THE WORKAHOLIC'S WORKOUT

It's 3:00 P.M. You've been working on a budget report since lunch, barely stopping while you've answered phone calls and e-mail messages. You're starting to feel that afternoon low coming on. Should you break to get a candy bar? Have your assistant get you a double espresso?

No. Get up. Shut your door. Turn out the light. Forward your calls to voice mail. Reboot your computer. Allot yourself 5 uninterrupted minutes, and try one of these hatha yoga poses that will give you a quick energy fix.

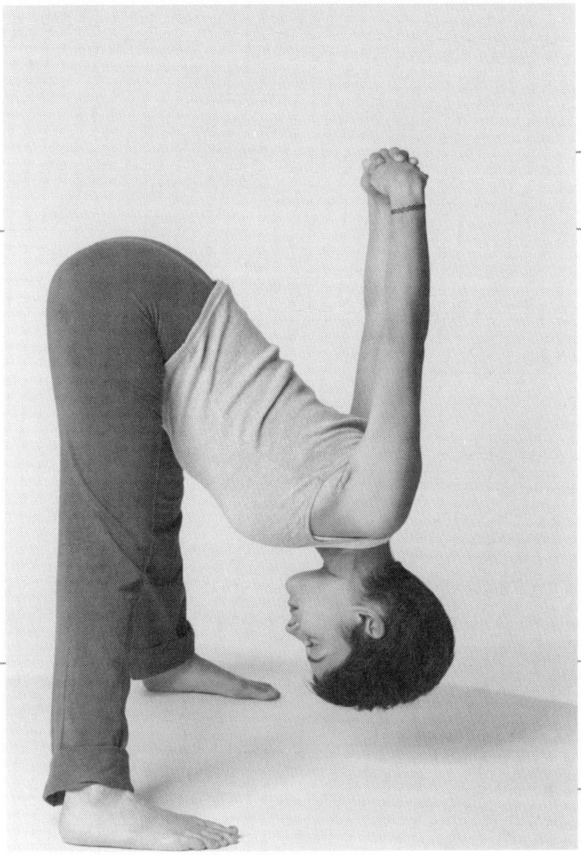

## STEP 3: LEARNING HOW TO RELAX

**Prasarita padottanasana (or wide-legged forward bend)**

This is a refreshing standing pose that opens the shoulders, lower back, and backs of the legs. It helps to counteract the rounding of your shoulders that you can get sitting in front of a computer all day.

Stand with your legs slightly wider than shoulder-width apart. Bend forward at your waist and raise your arms straight up over your head so that they are perpendicular to the floor.

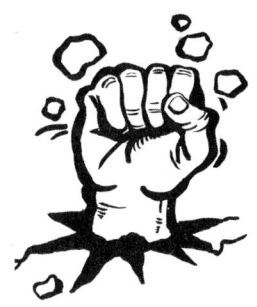

# THE WORKAHOLIC'S WORKOUT

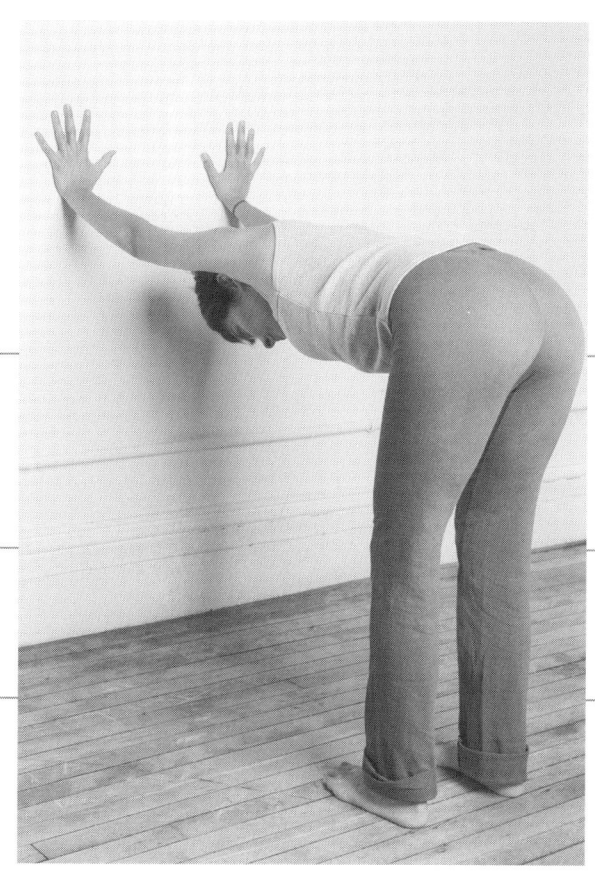

### Downward-facing dog (or hands-on-the-wall)

Put your hands on the wall and step back until you are in an L-shape. Your knees should be slightly bent. Your arms should be in line with your spine. Keep your back straight—do not arch it. Move your shoulder blades together and gently press your chest toward the floor. Feel the backs of your legs opening and your buttocks stretching. This pose is good for your lower back.

## STEP 3: LEARNING HOW TO RELAX

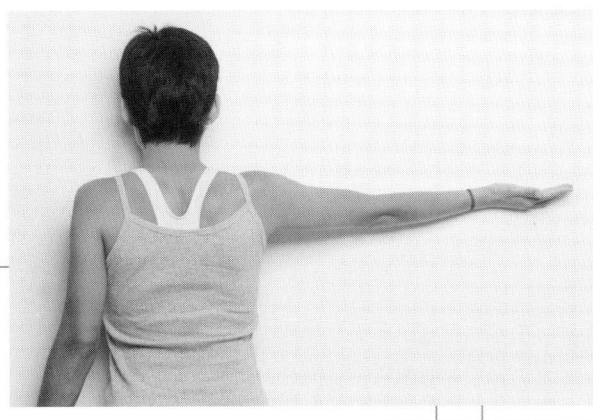

### Pectoral/front deltoid stretch

Even though your chest muscles, or pectorals, are in the front of the body, they tend to get tight when your shoulders are out of alignment from bending over a desk or computer.

Stand facing the wall. With palm facing up, stretch one arm out to the side along the wall. Turn slightly in the direction away from the hand. Do not arch your back—try to "broaden" it.

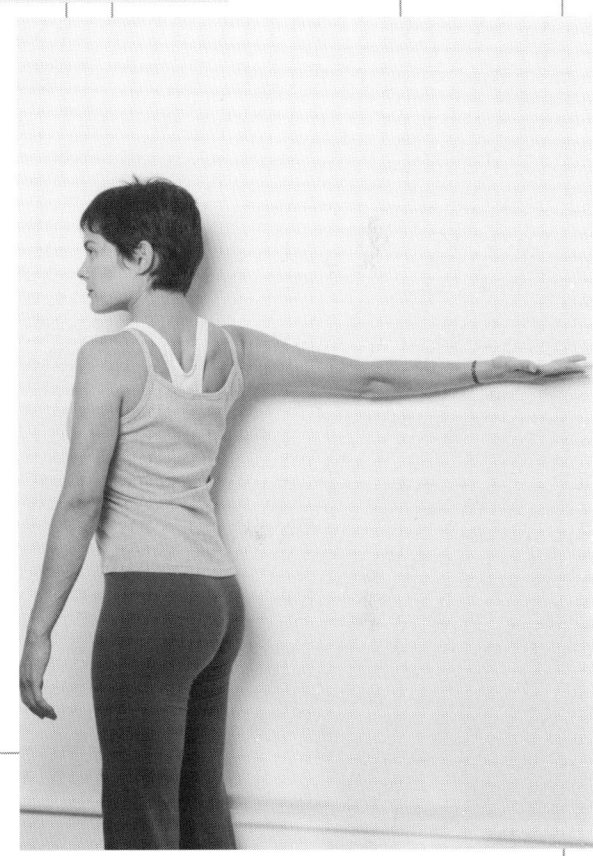

## LET SOMEONE ELSE WORK YOUR MUSCLES

Massage helps to stimulate blood flow to muscles, loosen tight muscles, relieve tension, and promote relaxation. It also helps to eliminate lactic acid, a chemical waste product that builds up in muscle tissue during exercise. Consider trying one of these three different types of massage:

1. Swedish massage is the most popular form of massage therapy. The therapist manipulates muscles lightly or deeply, depending on your comfort level.
2. While Swedish massage focuses on muscle manipulation, Shiatsu massage is energy oriented. The therapist locates and stimulates specific energy pressure points on the body. This increase of energy flow in the body assists the functioning of internal organs.
3. Reflexology focuses on loosening joints in the hands and feet to clear blockages along the energy meridians that lead to the body's vital organs.

OK, so you made it past 3:00 without loading up on sugar and caffeine. It's 7:00, and you're ready to leave the office. Your mind is still racing—will your boss approve your budget, should you call a client on the West Coast, how can you get in line for that promotion?

What's the first thing you do when you walk in the door? Open the fridge? Collapse on the couch and turn on the tube? Check your home e-mail?

Trying to force your mind to slow down will probably just perpetuate your agitation. Eating quickly, drinking alcohol, or going right to sleep only dulls the mind; it won't restore your vitality. Instead, try one of these poses that will calm you and help refocus your mind on the activities you want to do at home:

## STEP 3: LEARNING HOW TO RELAX

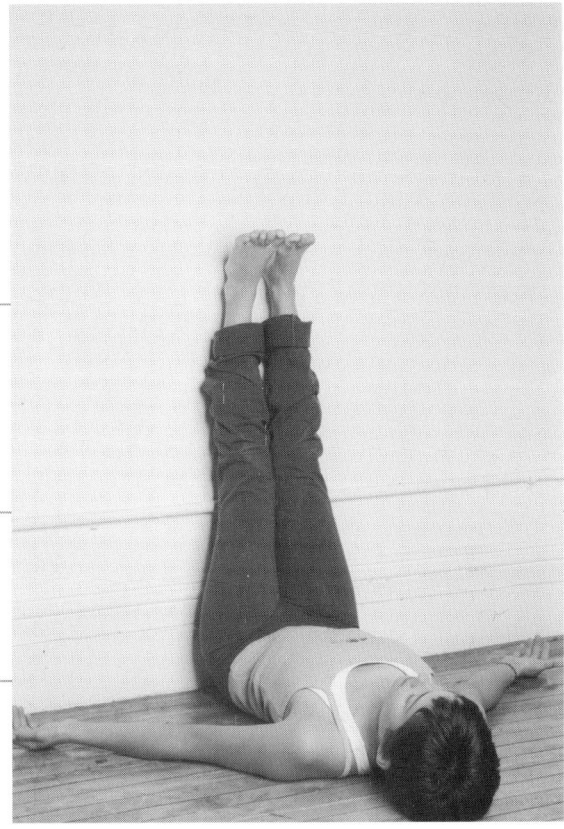

### Viparita Karani (or legs-up-the-wall)

Lie on the floor and put your feet up so that your heels rest against the wall. Putting your feet up reduces swelling and fatigue in the legs. It's OK to bend your knees if your lower back is sensitive. Your arms should be out to your sides. This pose is recommended for easing minor hypertension (which is currently being treated with medication). Hold this pose for 5 to 15 minutes. To come out of this pose, simply roll over to your right side.

# THE WORKAHOLIC'S WORKOUT

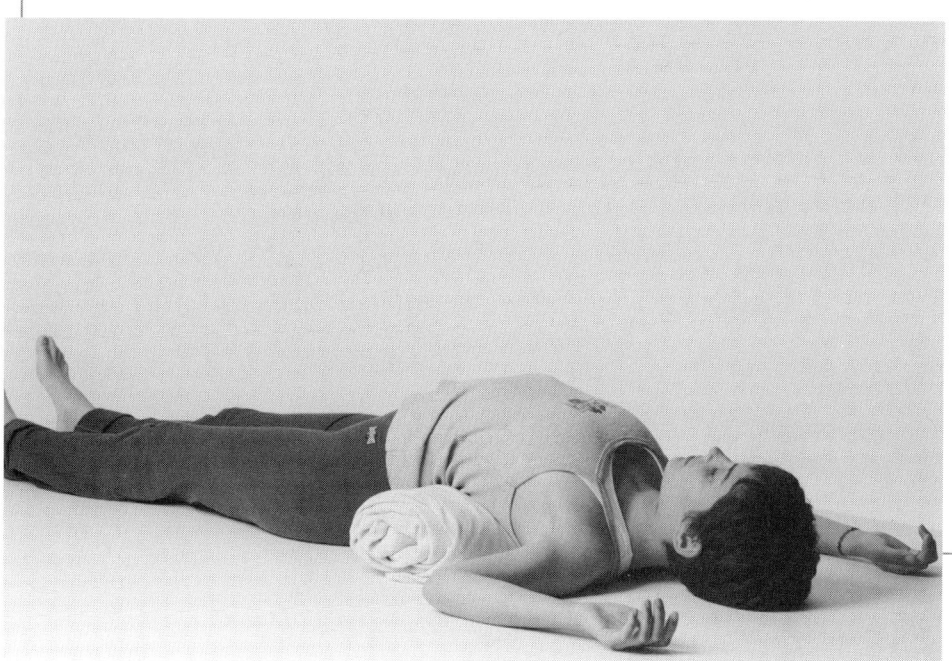

### Refreshing backbend

This pose opens your chest and shoulders—it's an antidote for our tendency toward the poor posture of rounding forward.

Lie on the floor and place a folded towel or blanket under your upper back, at the base of your shoulder blades. Your shoulders should touch the floor. Place your hands on the floor above your head.

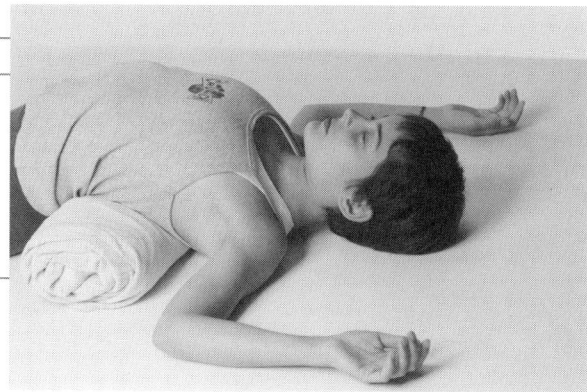

# STEP 3: LEARNING HOW TO RELAX

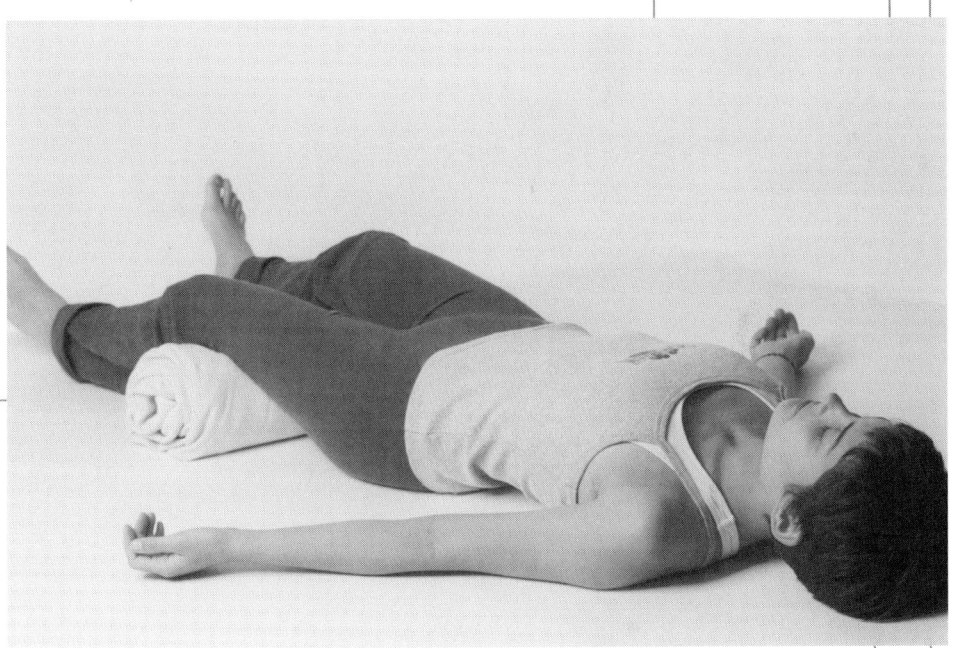

### Savasana

Place a rolled up blanket or towel under your knees and lie on the floor with your arms at your sides and palms open. Close your eyes. You can use an eye pillow to block out more light. Stay in this position for 5 to 15 minutes. This pose calms the mind, restores energy, and reduces physiological measures of stress, such as blood pressure, heart rate, and muscle tension.

# THE WORKAHOLIC'S WORKOUT

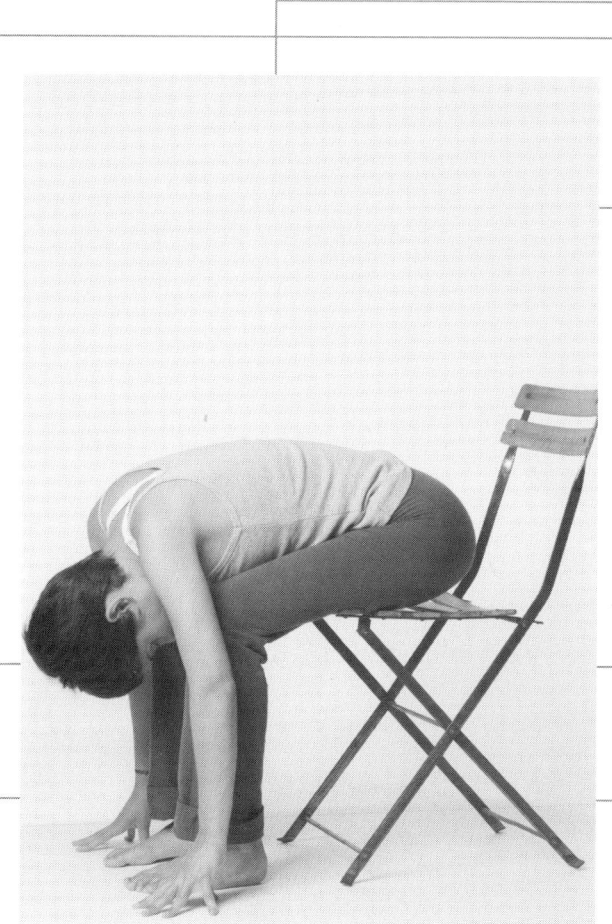

**Chair forward bend**

While sitting in your chair, just bend over your legs and rest for 3 minutes.

This pose stretches the lower back, relieves shoulder tension, and increases blood flow to your brain.

**STEP 3: LEARNING HOW TO RELAX**

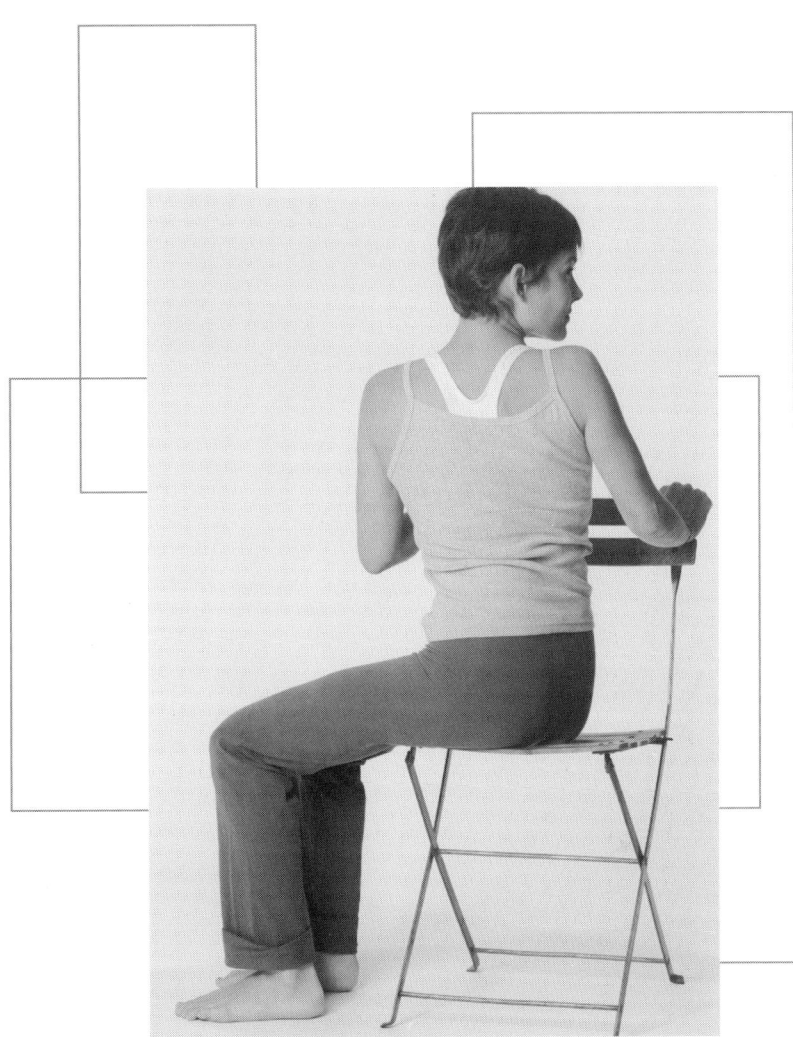

**Chair twists**

Sit sideways in your chair. Grab the back of the chair with your hands and turn your torso toward the back of the chair. Keep your back straight.

# THE WORKAHOLIC'S WORKOUT

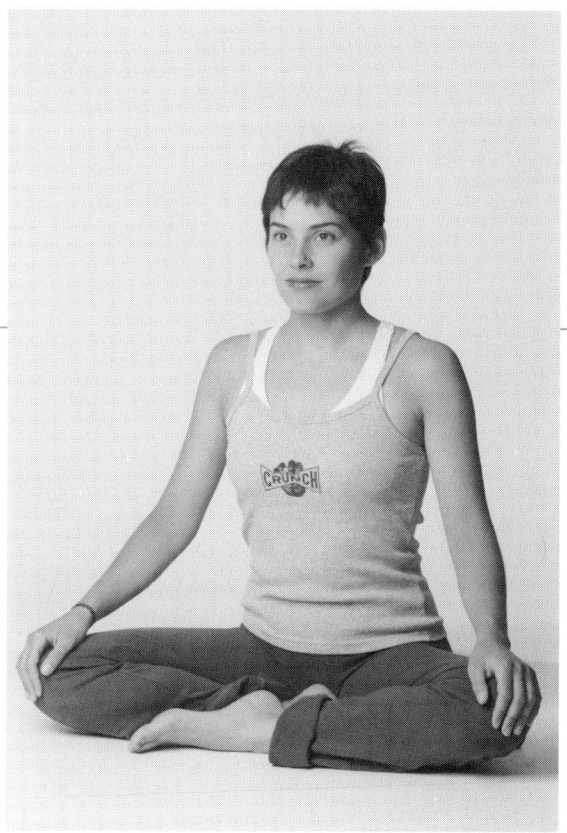

### Calming breath

Sit in a near lotus position. Close your eyes and take deep, rhythmic breaths. Focus on your breathing.

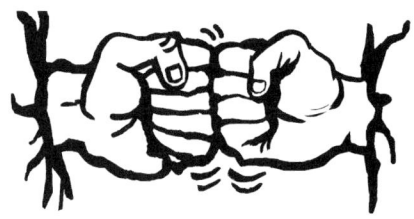

## STEP 3: LEARNING HOW TO RELAX

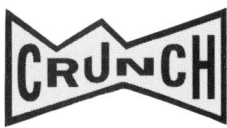

Yoga poses relieve tension in your muscles and help you clear your mind. You can hold a pose for a few seconds or for 15 minutes—however long you choose. While the physical aspects of yoga reduce stress and revitalize your body, yoga also has a spiritual component. People who are constantly busy working, traveling, and worrying often neglect the spiritual aspect of their lives. Yoga gives you a chance to rediscover it.

The following quote from yoga instructor John Friend captures the essence and purpose of hatha yoga poses:

> In their highest form, yoga postures (asanas) are joyful and loving celebrations of the inner Self. There are many metaphors for describing the inner Self, the spiritual essence inside each one of us described in the yoga scriptures. This essence has been called a spark of divinity or a luminous drop of divine consciousness that resides in the heart. Yoga is a means to reunite that little spark

with the cosmic flame, to merge that individual drop with the ocean of consciousness. When hatha yoga postures are performed with the fundamental intention of uniting with cosmic consciousness, the practice becomes spiritually uplifting. Each pose then becomes both a reflection of our yearning for this joyful reunion and a celebration of the immediate presence of this inner divinity.

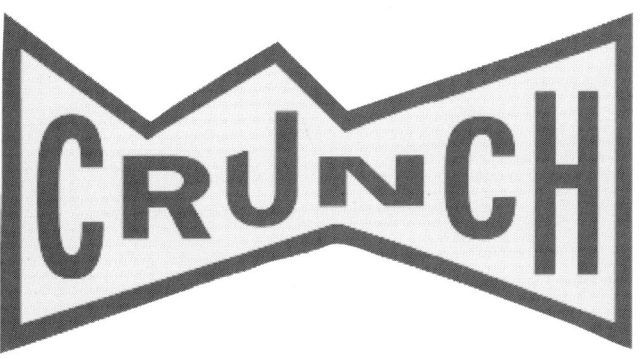

# PART IV
# STEP 4: EATING WELL

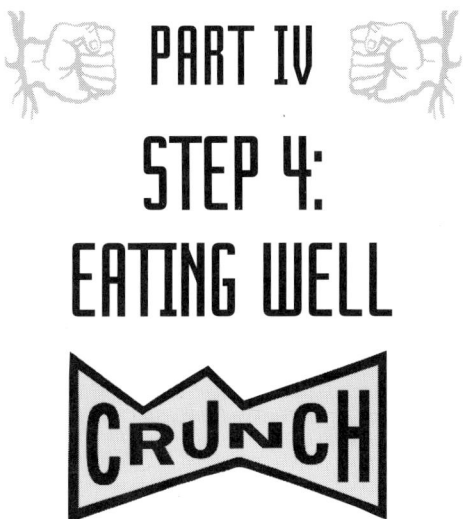

When you're stressed out and pressed for time, meals can be anything but nutritious. Workaholics are notorious breakfast-skippers, fast food junkies, caffeine swillers, and candy-bar snackers. Throw in the occasional rich, fat-laden business lunch, and is it any wonder your nerves are jangling, your waist is expanding, and you can't sleep at night despite feeling exhausted?

A nutritious, healthy diet alone can help energize you when you need energy and relax you when you need rest—and it's a whole lot easier than you think. If you spend a little time reading the following program now, you'll also find that eating well by sticking to the program is not nearly as time-consuming as typical calorie-counting, restrictive, fad diets.

At CRUNCH, we believe in combining working out with eating right. Most people know that eating too much can sabotage their fitness efforts, but it is also crucial to eat the correct kinds of foods. Without the proper nutrients in the right ratios, you could be holding your body back from reaching its fitness potential—and keeping your mind working at peak efficiency. All it takes to get the most out of your workouts, to lose body fat, and to gain muscle is to educate yourself on the facts.

At CRUNCH Los Angeles, Eatwize™ Program directors Larry Krug and Brian Blacher with Jennifer Nardini, head of research and development, are using years' worth of testing, research, and real-world experience to bring clients the Eatwize™ Program, an individually tailored fat loss plan that really works.

Before you begin, let's debunk a popular myth—that in order to lose weight, you need to exist on minute portions of food and feel completely miserable all the time. We Eatwize™ folks know that healthful eating isn't something to be dreaded or endured. Low-calorie, "crash" diets simply don't work. Period. Many clients come to us and swear that their friend lost weight on one of the high-protein, low-cal, high-carbohydrate, only fruit, no fruit, or any one of the myriad of diet trends out there today. The reality is that nearly all of the diets on the market at this time are just that—diets. They restrict calories to as low as 800 per day and offer the body up to all sorts of nutritional imbalances. This, coupled with the fact that any food plan that dips below 1,200 calories per day can cause your metabolism to slow down and hang on to your fat stores for dear life, makes most of these plans not only ineffective, but dangerous to your health.

Most weight lost on low-calorie diets, or any diet that causes you to lose more than two pounds a week, comes from water and muscle loss—not from fat. This is why so many people who claim to have lost weight on a crash diet regain it as soon as they have to start eating normally again. Plus, with less muscle and the same amount of fat, you won't be as toned or as energetic as you will be when you learn to eat more by eating "wize."

## GENERAL GUIDELINES

Five principles are essential to the Eatwise™ Program's high success rate. They are as follows:

**1. Aim for the 40-20-40 ratio.** Optimally, you should combine your daily carbohydrate, fat, and protein into a 40-20-40 ratio. This does not mean that every food or every meal has to be a perfect 40-20-40 split, as long as your body maintains the 40-20-40 ratio in your system throughout the day.

It isn't enough to simply eat a 40-20-40 split of carbohydrates, fat, and protein. The Eatwise™ Program is about eating carbohydrates, proteins, and fats that are natural, low glycemic, and contain as few additives, preservatives, and chemicals as possible. The program also helps you get the right amount of vitamins, minerals, and antioxidants every day. The program allows you to enjoy your food while you lose weight. It is easy to follow and can adapt to your continually changing world by giving you the ability to make smart food choices anywhere you go.

We use this ratio as opposed to the more common 40-30-30 ratio because people who work out need more protein. Thirty percent fat simply ends up being too much for most people, especially since there are so many hidden fats in foods that even when you aim for 30% you may end up getting more.

**2. Eat five small meals daily.** To further optimize weight loss, we recommend eating three main meals and two snacks throughout the day. Any excess calories from an overload at any one meal may be stored as fat, so breaking it up can help ensure you don't exceed your threshold. Giving your body something to digest every three to four hours will leave you feeling satisfied as it keeps your metabolism working at a high level, thereby burning more fat. (What's more, a mid-morning and mid-afternoon break will keep you mentally as well as physically energized for the work at hand.)

Eating carbohydrates, which are sugars, causes your pancreas to release insulin, which transports sugar out of the blood, which in turn decreases your blood sugar levels. Eating protein releases glucagon, which transports sugars into the blood, causing your blood sugar levels to rise.

When you eat carbohydrates that cause your blood sugars to rise quickly, lots of insulin is released to deal with the overload. Too much insulin in your bloodstream can cause those carbohydrate sugars to be stored as fat.

Keeping your blood sugar levels stable seems to allow more of your fat stores to be accessed for fuel. To maintain steady blood sugar levels, combine complex carbohydrates, healthy fats, and lean proteins at each meal, or throughout the day in the best ratio we've found—40-20-40.

**3. Eat fruits and vegetables.** You've heard it before and you'll hear it again: Fruits are God's gift to healthful eaters. They're loaded with cancer-fighting vitamins and minerals. They deliver sugar in the form of fructose, which is more slowly absorbed into the body when wrapped in the high fiber of most whole fruits. Though they are a healthy way to satisfy your sweet tooth, certain fruits do cause a quick sugar release. When following a fat-loss plan, it is best if you eat only one of these types of fruits a day, max. (Food lists are provided later.)

Vegetables are God's other gift. Many health professionals are continuing to realize the powerful medicinal value of plants, touting them as the prevention or cure for most of our diseases. Above and beyond their excellent vitamin and mineral status, vegetables naturally contain phytochemicals, substances that protect them from their own diseases and outside toxins. Diets high in vegetables are also high in fiber, meaning that you can eat until you're full and still have many, many calories to spare. In addition, fiber keeps your colon cleansed, which is especially important to help prevent colon cancer and other intestinal problems.

**4. Avoid saturated fat and refined and processed foods.** So many people trying to lose weight are terrified of the fat gram. They've been taught that once any fat passes their lips, it immediately makes a beeline to join its many friends hanging out on their thighs and love handles. What many people don't know, however, is that eating fat is actually an important part of dropping pounds. Fat intake causes your body to let go of stored fat more easily. When you restrict your dietary fat substantially, your body thinks it needs to save what it already has in the event of a famine. So, follow the Eatwise™ guidelines and get 20 percent of your total daily calories from fat. Just make sure it's healthy fat like olive, avocado, canola, or peanut oils. Saturated fat, or fats derived from meat and other animal sources, like butter and cheese, are where other, healthier fats got their bad rap. Saturated fats contain cholesterol, as do some vegetable oils like palm and coconut oil. There seems to be little reason to eat saturated fat—it can clog your arteries, cause cancer, and is easily stored in your body.

Refined and over-processed foods can also present major stumbling blocks on your road to a strong, lean body. For starters, they can cause a big insulin release that may add to your fat stores. Since most of these foods (anything made with white flour or refined sugar, like cake, cookies, non-whole grain bagels, white bread—even rice cakes!) have little to no fiber content, they don't fill you up, and they are usually high in calories. Nor do they give you the sustained energy of their healthier, high-fiber counterparts, so you are likely to crash and crave even more of these carbs. Many people who think they are addicted to refined carbs, sugars, and fats are really caught in a vicious cycle of high and low blood sugar. To find out how to get off the roller coaster, read on!

**5. Control your hormones.** It is only human to fail on a restrictive, low-calorie diet. Your brain produces all sorts of chemicals to try to force you to eat if it thinks you are starving—and those chemicals are almost impossible to ignore. So what one person might call a failure, we at CRUNCH call heeding the call of survival. So this time, using the program, you will learn to circumvent your hormonal reactions by placating them with the right food combinations in the right amounts. Here are some of the most common reactions that occur in your body every time you eat.

**Insulin.** When you ingest carbohydrates, the hormone insulin is released by your pancreas into your bloodstream. Insulin's primary function is to transport blood sugar from the blood to your muscles and liver. Whenever insulin is released, carbohydrates become the body's primary source of energy. If you don't happen to be using much energy at the time, however, high levels of insulin may cause carbohydrates to be stored as fats.

Excess insulin in your system causes blood sugar levels to drop, which can result in disturbances in thinking, mood, or energy. When your blood sugar falls too low, it stimulates your appetite to eat more sugar, which produces more insulin. High insulin levels can thus wreak havoc on the system. When you get caught in the cycle, the only way you can get your sugar levels up again is to eat more sugar.

You can break the carbohydrate cycle by eating the right amount of fat and protein in your daily diet and the right amount of unrefined or low-glycemic carbohydrates. With the correct combinations, you can regulate the body's insulin levels and reduce your previously out-of-control cravings.

**Glucagon.** The pancreas releases glucagon into the bloodstream as part of the digestive process. Glucagon has the opposite effect from insulin. It releases sugar from the muscle and liver back into the bloodstream. This helps to maintain and stabilize blood sugar levels and allows the body to release fat for energy.

Glucagon releases carbohydrates into the bloodstream to be broken down into calories. Glucagon is stimulated by protein, therefore it is important to eat protein with carbohydrates to keep insulin and glucagon levels in balance. This is one reason the 40-20-40 ratio works so well.

**The glycemic index.** The glycemic index is a scale that rates how fast food becomes glucose in your bloodstream and therefore how much insulin is secreted to help metabolize that food. If a food has a low glycemic index, less insulin is released and the amount of glucose derived from that food is sustained in the bloodstream over a longer period of time. This is a good thing, because stable blood sugar means less fat stored and more released.

Food with a high glycemic index causes the release of more insulin more rapidly. The glucose will last for a shorter period of time, which in turn may cause you to become hungry more quickly, and you'll run out of energy faster.

## THE EATWIZE™ PRINCIPLES FOR EATING OUT

- Avoid eating the bread when it is brought to the table.
- Have a small snack before going to a restaurant in case it takes a while before you get your food.
- Consider splitting your meal with somebody—many restaurants serve very large portions.
- Order salads with dressing on the side.
- Do not order cream-based foods.
- Tell the server exactly how you want your food prepared.
- Always share your dessert if you decide to order one.
- Asked for steamed veggies, not sautéed.
- Save your member C foods for when you eat out, when you always have less control.

Lucky for you, we've removed the guesswork for you. Our food lists show you clearly which foods you can indulge in and which you should eat in moderation. In order to maximize weight loss, always aim for the low glycemic foods. (Note: We have rated our food choices by other factors, such as how natural it is, and how many sugars, additives, and preservatives it contains. Not all "free" foods for are completely low glycemic, but they may have other redeeming properties that make them perfectly acceptable choices).

## HOW TO MAKE SENSE OF FOOD LABELS

Here's more guesswork out the window, courtesy of Eatwize™. When beginning a new eating plan, it's smart to stock your personal space at home or work with healthful foods you can easily prepare. Here's a breakdown on how to read a standard food label, as well as a breakdown of the terminology.

Consider this example of a label of 2% low-fat milk:

### Nutrition Facts

| | |
|---|---|
| Serving size | 1 cup (240ml) |
| Servings per container | about 2 |

Percent daily values are based on a 2,000 calorie diet. Your daily values may be higher or lower based on your caloric needs.

## STEP 4: EATING WELL

|  | Amount per serving | % daily value |
|---|---|---|
| Calories | 130 | |
| Calories from fat | 45 | |
| Total fat | 5 g | 8 % |
| Saturated fat | 3 g | 5 % |
| Cholesterol | 2 mg | 8 % |
| Sodium | 130 mg | 5 % |
| Total Carbohydrates | 13 g | 4 % |
| Dietary fiber | 0 g | 0 % |
| Sugars | 13 g | |
| Protein | 10 g | 19 % |
| Vitamin A | | 10 % |
| Vitamin C | | 4 % |
| Calcium | | 35 % |
| Iron | | 0 % |
| Vitamin D | | 25 % |

The above figures are based on the caloric needs of a person on a 2,000 calorie-a-day diet. Here are the needs of a 2,500 calorie-a-day diet, for comparison:

| Calories | 2,000 | 2,500 |
|---|---|---|
| Total fat | less than 6 g | 80 g |
| Saturated fat | less than 20 g | 25 g |
| Cholesterol | less than 30 mg | 300 mg |
| Sodium | less than 2,400 mg | 2,400 mg |
| Total Carbohydrates | less than 300 g | 375 g |
| Dietary Fiber | 25 g | 30 g |
| Protein | 50 g | 65 g |

1. Look at the serving size (1 cup).
2. Check to see how many servings are in the container (2 servings).
3. See how many calories are in the serving (130 calories).
4. Look how many calories are from fat (45 calories).
5. Determine the percentage of total calories coming from fat. The maximum calories from fat should not exceed 20%. Calories from fat divided by total calories per serving is equal to the percentage of calories coming from fat. If this percentage is more than 20% there is too much fat (45 divided by 130 = 32%).
6. Don't be fooled by the percentages given in the right hand column. Those numbers refer to the Recommended Daily Allowances. For example, in 2% fat milk, the calories from fat are not 2% of the total calories, but 32%. Check to see how much fat and what type of fat is in the product.

7. See how much sugar is in the product. On this label, all 13 grams of carbohydrates are pure sugar.

Fat-free labels are usually high in sugar and chemicals, and unfortunately, fat-free does not mean calorie-free. Sugar is often substituted for taste instead of fat.

Did you know that a food can be labeled calorie-free and still have calories? According to the American Heart Association, the following criteria must be met when making certain claims about food:

- Calorie-Free: fewer than 5 calories.
- Light (Lite): One-third fewer calories, or no more than half the fat or sodium of the regular versions.
- Fat-Free: less than 0.5 gram of fat.
- Low Fat: no more than 3 grams of fat.
- Reduced or Less Fat: at least 25% less fat.
- Lean: less than 10 grams of fat, 4 grams of saturated fat, and 95 mg of cholesterol.
- Extra Lean: less than 5 grams of fat, 2 grams, and 95 mg. of cholesterol.
- Low in Saturated Fat: no more than 1 gram of fat and 15% of calories from saturated fat.
- Cholesterol Free: less than 2 mg. cholesterol and 2 grams of saturated fat.
- Low Cholesterol: no more than 20 mg. of cholesterol and 2 grams of saturated fat.
- Reduced Cholesterol: at least 25% less cholesterol and 2 grams or less of saturated fat.
- Sodium Free: fewer than 5 mg. of sodium and no sodium chloride.
- Very Low Sodium: 35 or fewer mg. of sodium.
- Low Sodium: no more than 140 mg. of sodium.
- Reduced or Less Sodium: at least 25% less sodium.
- Sugar Free: less than 0.5 gram of sugar.
- No added sugar: means no added sucrose—however, it could mean that the food is sweetened with honey, syrups, or fruit juice.
- Low Sugar: Less than 5% of total weight.
- Unsweetened fruit juice may have no added sugar, but fruit juice *is* sugar.
- Sugar free, fat free, dairy free: If the product is sugar free, fat free, dairy free, taste free etc., it does not mean it is calorie free—it will still have carbohydrates or protein.
- High Fiber: at least 5 grams of fiber.
- Good Source of Fiber: 2.5 to 4.9 grams of fiber.

## STEP 4: EATING WELL

On the first day of the following program, write down your starting weight and body fat percentage. You can have a personal trainer or a nutritionist test your body fat, or go to your local gym if you're unfamiliar with the process. Then, record your new, improved stats once a week.

Within six months you can expect to lose anywhere from five to 25 pounds of fat, or 10 to 15% total. Of course, the amount you lose may vary from what other people experience, based on your current body composition, activity level, and genetic factors. Obviously, the more closely you stick to the plan, the better your results will be.

## FREE VEGETABLES

Feel free to have as many of these veggies as you like without counting them toward your daily calorie totals.

| | | |
|---|---|---|
| Arame | Collard Greens | Peppers |
| Artichokes | Cucumber | Radishes |
| Arugula | Dulse | Rhubarb |
| Asparagus | Eggplant | Rutabaga |
| Bamboo Shoots | Endives | Scallions |
| Beetroot | Green Beans | Spinach |
| Bok Choy | Jicama | Sprouts |
| Broccoli | Kale | Swiss Chard |
| Cabbage | Kelp | Tomatoes |
| Cauliflower | Lettuce | Turnips |
| Celery | Kohlrabi | Water Chestnuts |
| Chicory | Mushroom | Watercress |
| Chives | Onions | Zucchini |

## FREE FOODS

These are foods you can also have in moderation without counting them as part of your daily intake:

| **Condiments** | **Drinks** |
|---|---|
| Anchovelle Paste | Coffee* |
| Ketchup | Tea* |
| Garlic | Herbal Tea |
| Horseradish | Wheatgrass Juice |
| Lemon Juice | Diet Soda* |
| Mint | Non Caloric Drinks |

# THE WORKAHOLIC'S WORKOUT

**Condiments** (continued)
Ginger
Mustard
Salsa
Soy Sauce (light)
Spices
Tamarind
Tobasco
Vinegar
Wasabi

**Foods**
Diet Jell-O
Non-Calorie Foods
Cucumbers (pickled)

*Not more than one cup a day

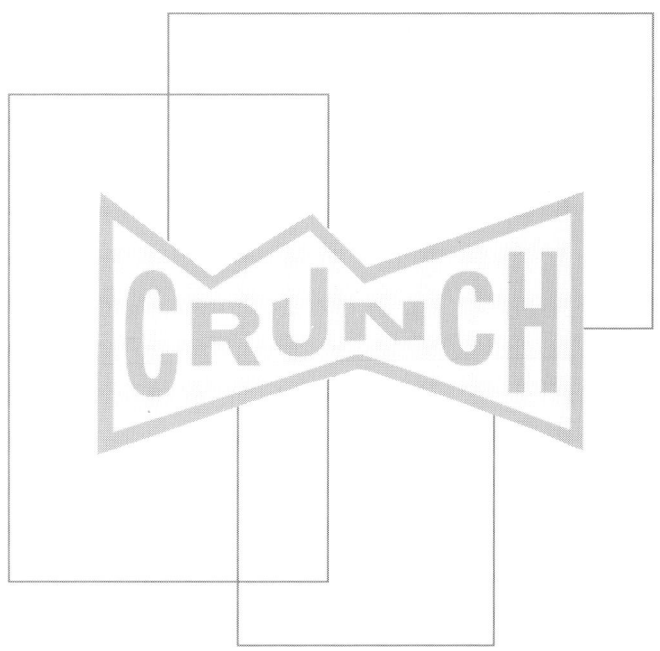

## STEP 4: EATING WELL

# THE SIX-MONTH PLAN

|  | Women | Men |
|---|---|---|
| Calories: | 1,200 to 1,400 | 1,400 to 1,800 |
| Carbohydrates: | 4 to 5 medium-size servings per day. (approx. 100 calories) | 6 to 7 servings per day |
| Fats: | 2 servings per day | 3 servings per day |
| Protein: | 4 to 5 servings per day | 5 to 6 serving daily |

## Carbohydrate list:

*A small serving (3 oz.) of:*

Apple, Apricots, Barley, Berries, Cereal (high fiber, no sugar), Cherries, Grapefruit, Guava, Lentils, Oatmeal, Peas, Plums, Pumpkin, Rice (brown, basmati), Squash, Strawberries, Sweet Potatoes, Tangerine, Vegetable Garden Burger

The carbs listed above have the lowest glycemic rating, the lowest amounts of sugar and are the least refined and processed. When choosing from the following carbs, which are higher on the glycemic index, do not exceed 5 servings a day:

Bananas, Bread (high fiber, low sugar), Buckwheat, Bulgar Wheat, Cereal (high-fiber, low-sugar), Corn, Cous-Cous, Fruit Salad (citrus, no sugar), Fruit Snacks (dried, no sugar), Grapes, Grits, Honey, Kiwi, Nectarine, Noodles (soba and udon), Oat Bran (hot cereal).

*Do not exceed 1 serving per day of:*

Applesauce (non-sugar), Bagel, Baguette, Beer (light or regular), White Bread/Roll/Pita, Canned Fruit (non-sugar) , Cantaloupe, Carrot Juice, Carrots, Cereal (low sugar), Chips (low fat), Cornstarch, Crackers (salty), Crackers/Cookies (sweet), Cream of Wheat, Croissant/Muffin, Croutons, Dried Fruit (mixed), Figs, Flour (all), Frozen Yogurt (nonfat), Fruit Juice (all).

# THE WORKAHOLIC'S WORKOUT

## Fat list

*A small serving (3 oz.) of:*

Avocado, Nuts (all), Oils (olive, canola, flaxseed sesame, soybean), Olives, Pumpkin Seeds.

The fats listed above are unsaturated, and by consuming *only* those fats for your 20% daily fat allowance, you will lose weight more quickly than if you also choose from among the following fats:

Coconut, Guacamole, Humus, Oil (corn, peanut, sunflower), Nut Butters (almond, cashew, etc.), Peanut Butter (light, natural), Salad Dressing (low fat, no cream), Sesame Seeds, Sunflower Seeds.

*Do not exceed 1 serving per day of:*

Butter, Dips (cream-based), Margarine, Marinades, BBQ Sauces, Mayonnaise (light), Palm Oil, Pesto Sauce, Salad Dressing (low fat, cream).

## Protein list:

*A small serving (3 oz.) of:*

Chicken Breast, Egg, Egg Whites, Fish (white fish), Protein Powders (all), Soya Burger (fat free), Tofu (low fat, low sodium), Tuna (canned, white, in water),Turkey Breast (white meat)

The proteins above are the highest quality of protein with the least amount of saturated bad fats. If you choose from among the following protein list, do not exceed 5 servings per day:

Cottage Cheese (low fat), Cottage Cheese (fat free), Fish (pink), Hot Dog (tofu, fat-free), Vegetarian Protein Burger, Ground Turkey (97% lean), Scallops, Shrimp, Prawns, Oysters, Turkey Slice (fat free).

*Do not exceed 1 serving per day of:*

Beef (93% lean ground), Beef Burger, Beef Steak (lean), Sirloin Fillet, Cold Cut (lean), Duck, Lamb, Pork.

Keep track of your progress with the following chart:

| Week | Date | Weight (lbs.) | Body fat % | Fat loss in % | Weight loss (in lbs.) |
|---|---|---|---|---|---|
| 1 | | | | | |
| 2 | | | | | |
| 3 | | | | | |
| etc. | | | | | |

## STEP 4: EATING WELL

## IT'S JUST A NUMBER

You really can't tell much from staring at the numbers on the scale. They can't tell you how much of your total weight comes from fat, muscle, bone, or water. Only a professional fat percentage or body composition test can tell you that. It is possible to lose fat, gain muscle, drop a dress size, feel and look great, and still gain weight! Muscle weighs more per area than fat does, so make certain that you look to your body fat testing for the real scoop on your progress. To help you decode the numbers you'll get back, here is a chart of body-fat ranges.

## MALES (% BODY FAT)

| Age | Excellent | Very Good | Good | Average | Fair | Poor |
|---|---|---|---|---|---|---|
| 19–24 | 6–10 | 11–13 | 14–17 | 18–21 | 22–25 | > 25 |
| 25–29 | 6–10 | 11–14 | 15–18 | 19–22 | 23–26 | > 26 |
| 30–34 | 6–10 | 11–15 | 16–19 | 20–23 | 24–27 | > 27 |
| 35–39 | 6–10 | 11–16 | 17–20 | 21–24 | 25–28 | > 28 |
| 40–44 | 6–10 | 11–17 | 18–21 | 22–25 | 26–29 | > 29 |
| 45–49 | 6–10 | 11–18 | 19–22 | 23–26 | 27–30 | > 30 |
| 50+ | 6–10 | 11–19 | 20–23 | 24–27 | 28–31 | > 31 |

## FEMALES (% BODY FAT)

| Age | Excellent | Very Good | Good | Average | Fair | Poor |
|---|---|---|---|---|---|---|
| 18–24 | 8–12 | 13–15 | 16–19 | 20–23 | 24–27 | > 27 |
| 25–29 | 8–12 | 13–16 | 17–20 | 21–24 | 25–28 | > 28 |
| 30–34 | 8–12 | 13–17 | 18–21 | 22–25 | 26–29 | > 29 |
| 35–39 | 8–12 | 13–18 | 19–22 | 23–26 | 27–30 | > 30 |
| 40–44 | 8–12 | 13–19 | 20–23 | 24–27 | 28–31 | > 31 |
| 45–49 | 8–12 | 13–20 | 21–24 | 25–28 | 29–32 | > 32 |
| 50+ | 8–12 | 13–21 | 22–25 | 26–29 | 30–33 | > 33 |

## MAINTENANCE

It's certainly possible to eat healthy meals and lose weight while maintaining an active, busy lifestyle. Once you see how much difference finding an eating program that compliments your workouts can make, you'll probably want to make it a permanent addition to your life.

## THE WORKAHOLIC'S WORKOUT

Please consult your physician before starting any nutritional program. This is only part of the Eatwize™ Program—log onto **www.eatwize.com** for more information.

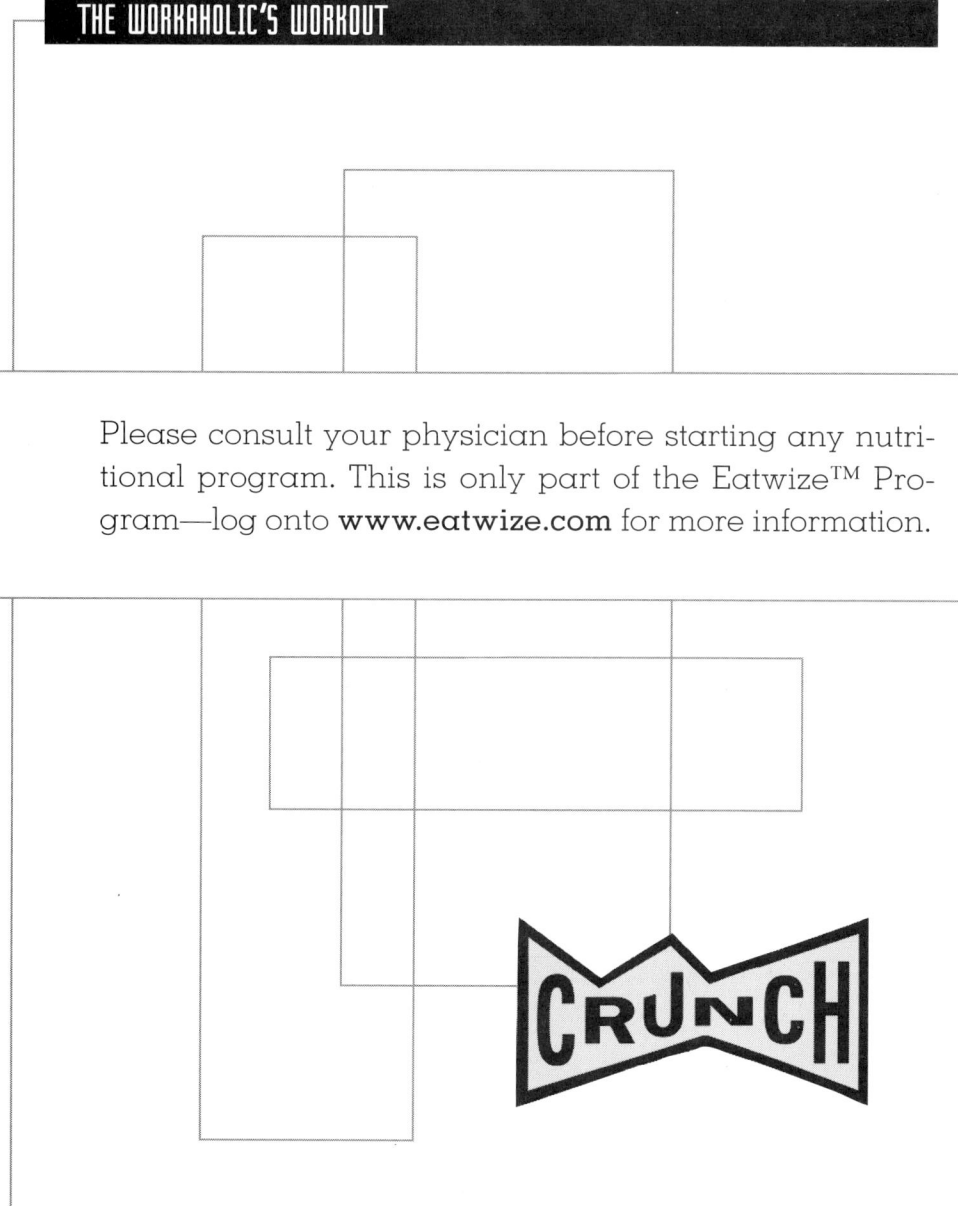

# PART V
# STEP 5: COMBATING STRESS

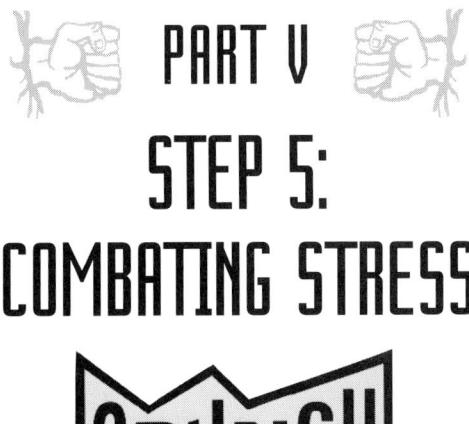

As we discussed in Part 1, there are two types of workaholics: those who work excessively by choice and those who work excessively because they feel they have no choice.

The first type of workaholic loves her work, thrives on it, and throws herself into it with utter passion. The second type may work excessively out of fear of losing his job or anxiety about pleasing a boss and "measuring up." This second type of workaholic may also spend an inordinate amount of time at work simply in order to avoid stressful situations in his personal life. It is this second type of workaholic that suffers the most from stress.

Stress is one of those catchall words that are hard to define. Stress can have physical sources, emotional sources, or mental sources: You can "get stressed" running errands all day or just sitting at your desk trying to prepare a budget—or even having a confrontational run-in at the water cooler with a difficult co-worker. Deadlines and other time pressures are usually a big factor in creating stress.

While no one can completely avoid stress, we can all learn to handle it well so that it doesn't become a chronic condition. Living under constant stress, experiencing relentless anxiety and muscular tension, can lead to serious physical and mental illnesses.

As we've described, exercising, eating well, and getting enough sleep all help reduce stress. Having a positive mental outlook, even during trying times, is also a key factor in combating stress. Being an optimist is easier said than done, however. When you feel anxious

## THE WORKAHOLIC'S WORKOUT

### COMMON SOURCES OF STRESS IN THE WORKPLACE

- Not being sure what you're expected to do in your job
- Being afraid you may lose your job
- Confusing the nature of your relationships with your boss, co-workers, subordinates because of "ghosts"—like reacting to a boss the way you did a parent or imagining intense competition between yourself and co-workers because that's what you were exposed to in the past
- Very real problems with a boss—e.g., one who never praises, always criticizes, doesn't make your responsibilities clear, is poorly organized but expects you to make up for his or her deficiencies
- Co-workers who are competitive to the point of undermining your efforts
- Subordinates who don't carry their weight for whatever reason
- Financial problems within the organization or company
- Trickle-down bad management
- Failure to be properly prepared for significant changes within the organization
- Disparity of values—yours vs. the company's, such as fundamentally objecting to products that damage people's health or the environment
- Poor communications
- Major changes in management, structure, operations, staff, location

Source: *Take Command: Career & Achievement*, The Hatherleigh Company, Ltd.

and overwhelmed by stress, take a few moments to put your situation in perspective. Remind yourself how you got through difficult times in the past. Think about your accomplishments and the friends and family who have stood by you over the years.

Dr. Frederic Flach, psychiatrist and author of *Resilience: The Power to Bounce Back When the Going Gets Tough*, believes that the key to overcoming stress is to jumpstart your creativity. By applying some creative problem-solving techniques to one stressful situation, he argues, you will become more resilient and better able to handle the next stressful situation that (inevitably) comes along. We're all creative to some degree—the more we tap our creative abilities, the better we adapt to, or overcome, stress. Behavioral scientists have drawn

## STEP 5: COMBATING STRESS

conclusions about the attributes of the creative personality that are particularly relevant to resilience. For example, by using standardized psychological tests to identify personality traits commonly associated with a high degree of skill at creative problem solving, scientists have shown that people who are good at looking at old problems in new ways, coming up with new options, and choosing the most suitable and workable solutions to various dilemmas also seem best able to deal with challenge and sustain or restore personal coherence under stressful conditions. The more creative a person is, the more likely he is to be independent in thought and action; possess a strong, but supple, sense of self-esteem; be receptive to new ideas; exhibit a wide range of interests; tolerate uncertainty and distress for a prolonged, though reasonable, length of time; enjoy mystery as much as definitiveness; and commit himself to life, his work, and the people with whom he is involved within the framework of a meaningful philosophy of life.

In addition to creativity, resilient people also tend to possess the following attributes:

- A strong, supple sense of self-esteem
- Independence of thought and action, without fear of relying on others or reluctance to do so
- The ability to give and take in one's interactions with others, and a well-established network of personal friends, including one or more who serve as confidants
- A high level of personal discipline and a sense of responsibility
- Recognition and development of one's special gifts and talents
- Open-mindedness and receptivity to new ideas
- A willingness to dream
- A wide range of interests
- A keen sense of humor
- Insight into one's own feelings and those of others, and the ability to communicate these in an appropriate manner
- A high tolerance of distress
- Focus, a commitment to life, and a philosophical framework within which personal experiences can be interpreted with meaning and hope, even at life's seemingly most hopeless moments

The caveat for any such list of wonderful traits is, of course, that none of us is perfect. We are always more or less any one of these things: a little weak on self-esteem, perhaps, but quite open to new ideas; enjoying a wide range of interests, but having trouble focusing on one or two to develop more fully; gifted with a sense of humor, but so tolerant of distress that we put up with unhealthy, demeaning, even abusive behavior in others for much too long a time; willing to dream of what we wish to accomplish with our lives, but finding it hard to muster up the self-discipline required to take the often arduous steps to realize our dreams.

The ability to think and act creatively is a universal human strength. Of course, there are differences in the creative potential that each of us possesses, as well as in the degree to which we have developed this potential. There is also considerable difference with regard to the extent to which we are able to integrate creativity with other essential ingredients of resilience, such as the ability to tolerate distress and the discipline to pursue well-defined goals.

Nonetheless, the more we master creative problem-solving skills the more we will be able to respond to stressful situations resiliently. At first, our efforts to employ creative tactics may seem labored, even artificial. But with practice, these can become a basic part of our spontaneous response to challenge.

## STAGES IN THE CREATIVE PROBLEM-SOLVING PROCESS

Creative problem solving takes place in five stages, says Dr. Flach, which involve a delicate blending of logical and illogical thought processes. These stages vary in length and intensity with the issues that confront us. They do not always have to follow each other in strict sequence. Sometimes, a particular stage may require considerable

### TIPS FOR ADAPTING TO CHANGE IN THE WORKPLACE

- Don't let anxiety and insecurity get the best of you.
- Reach out to be as informed as you can be about changes that have occurred or are about to take place.
- Think carefully about how you and your responsibilities will be affected by the changes.
- Talk with your superiors and ask for guidance if you feel it would be helpful.
- Don't take things too personally.
- Be prepared to learn new skills.
- Try to understand how the changes will benefit the organization and how they may benefit you too.

Source: *Take Command: Career & Achievement*, The Hatherleigh Company, Ltd.

time and thought; other times, you can move through the stage with lightening speed.

1. The first stage is **fact-finding**. Here, you reexamine the situation to gain as much information about it as possible. Any significant life problem deserves such attention, whether the question is what career direction to choose, why you are single when getting married and having a family has always been a goal, how to renew a troubled marriage, or what to do with yourself after retirement.

2. The second is **problem finding**, in which you redefine issues, trying to see them in a new light. For example, a problem in deciding on a career path may really be rooted in an inability to divorce yourself from parental expectations; marriage conflicts may stem more from a failure to handle the demoralizing influence of in-laws than from the quality of the relationship with your spouse.

3. The next stage is **idea finding**. Here, you generate options based on your new view of the problem. For example, having explored the question of why you're not married and redefined the issue as a fear of intimacy, you can begin to think of new ways to improve your ability to relate to others—participating in group events, developing recreational interests such as skiing or tennis that can be shared with others, attending courses to develop self-confidence and social skills. Or, if the question of what to do after retirement has been redefined as what interests you had as an adolescent or young adult and have neglected in the years since, you can look back to those earlier times for valuable ideas.

4. The fourth stage is **solution finding**, in which you evaluate the meaning and both the positive and the negative consequences of the ideas you've produced. Now you are moving back to a more logical appraisal of options. Skiing and playing tennis might bring you in contact with more people and increase your chances of meeting someone special; however, if you're not that competitive, skiing would seem to be the better choice of the two. Moreover, since the real problem appears to be a fear of closeness, an encounter group experience or counseling would seem to be the most relevant course to pursue early on. Or again, having recognized that the negative effect of in-laws has been disrupting your marriage, and having considered a variety of ideas that range from belligerent confrontation to total avoidance, you may decide that the best course of action seems to be a heart-to-heart talk with your spouse to shape a "foreign policy" to deal with the relatives jointly and more effectively.

5. The final stage is **acceptance finding**, wherein you develop the best ideas as fully as possible and proceed to test them in the real world. Here, planning, initiative, and self-discipline are called into play.

## TWO CRITICAL GUIDELINES

Two vital guidelines for creative problem solving apply to each stage in the process, but most of us ignore or violate them regularly. They are the rule of deferred judgment and the rule that quantity leads to quality. It goes against the grain to withhold premature criticism during our search for ideas and to try to come up with as many ideas as we can. These two tactics, however, are important, as the ideas we come up with at first will usually be more stereotyped than those that emerge later on and afford us little by way of new insights. We all tend to jump in and analyze and criticize our own (as well as others') ideas as soon as they have been expressed. We have a natural tendency to limit the solutions we think of to a pitiful few. How about taking a vacation without the children, for example? "Not enough money. Besides, there's no one to take care of the kids." How about finding a way to facilitate a promotion in the company? "There's no point in even trying. It's all politics anyway." While the negatives may have a kernel of truth in them, bringing them up, one by one, as each new idea appears, automatically blocks the entrance of new, better, and more suitable options.

With few exceptions, we are all somewhat subject to the pressures of conformity, caught up in our present perception of reality, which has been formed and protected by habit and experience. We all fear new ideas that are too far out of the ordinary. We don't want to seem foolish, even if only to ourselves. Those of us with a long-standing vested interest in being out of the mainstream of thinking and behavior are no exception—we, too, can be thwarted in our creative efforts by an unimaginative adherence to nonconformity.

Keeping in mind these two particularly important rules—to defer judging solutions and to try to come up with as many solutions as possible, no matter how silly they may seem at first—we will increase our chances of seeing things in a new light and get in touch with the valuable resources of our unconscious.

## PUTTING STRESS INTO PERSPECTIVE

For the vast majority of the world's population, work of any kind is often a matter of life or death—scratching at dry earth in a desperate

## STEP 5: COMBATING STRESS

### TIPS FOR REDUCING STRESS IN THE WORKPLACE

- Know your job as well as you possibly can.
- Go that extra mile; put in the effort and time needed to do your best.
- Be a source of positive input to your managers, co-workers, and subordinates. This includes everything from a smile and friendliness to praise, constructive criticism, honest communication, and enthusiasm.
- Be in command of your relationships at work. Deal with people as they really are, not colored by distortions.
- Keep a proper balance between your personal life and your work life. Render unto work what belongs at work and unto your personal life whatever belongs there. If you have problems at home, try to leave them there. If you have problems at work, don't make the people in the rest of your life suffer needlessly because of them.
- Get involved. If you're engaged in various activities and functions at work, you'll be better informed and, chances are, a lot more respected, too.
- Share the credit.
- Be organized.
- Commit yourself to excellence in the task at hand.
- Lead a balanced life: don't overdo it. Plan vacations.

Source: *Take Command: Career & Achievement*, The Hatherleigh Company, Ltd.

attempt to grow food, being paid in pennies to slave in front of machines to produce cloth materials that will eventually be shaped into fashionable designs and sold for hundreds of dollars in Paris.

Here in America we enjoy the unique luxury of choice. Never in history has a society offered so many people the privilege to choose the work they do. Yet how often do we make good career choices? How often do we feel trapped by our job or financial circumstances? The best job is one that gives us the opportunity to put into play our basic talents. We all have such talents, whether they are as simple as sewing a hem or as complex as higher mathematics or nuclear physics. We can find clues to these talents by looking back to childhood and adolescence and asking ourselves what sorts of activities we selected spontaneously to immerse ourselves in. Play is an important barometer: Did we, for example, enjoy spending time by ourselves, building model airplanes, collecting stamps, reading? Or did we pre-

## THE WORKAHOLIC'S WORKOUT

# SELF-ASSESSMENT FOR STRESS

Take a moment and evaluate your work environment for its strengths and weaknesses. Plan to improve areas of concern. Manage stress by addressing these issues energetically.

**The product or service**
- Does it fit into your value system?
- Is it good for people?
- Are you proud of it?

**The tasks**
- Do you like what you do?
- Is it meaningful?
- Do you do it (them) well?
- Do you need extra training?

**The people**
- Do you respect your manager(s)?
- Do they share your values?
- Are they a source of encouragement?
- Do they value your contributions?
- Do they manage well?
- Do you enjoy your co-workers?
- Do they do their jobs well?
- Do your subordinates perform well?
- Are you having difficulties with one person in particular?

**The office environment**
- Is it friendly? Attractive?
- Is safety emphasized?
- Do you feel good being there?
- Is there a sense of accomplishment?

**Other issues**
- Are you working too many hours?
- Are you adequately paid?
- Do you have the benefits you need?
- Is there a good system of job performance appraisal?
- Are you given enough responsibility?
- Are you given enough supervision?
- Are there opportunities for growth and promotion?
- Can you keep a consistent energy level?
- Do you exercise regularly?
- Have you taken a vacation recently?
- Do you plan to take a vacation in the near future?

Source: *Take Command: Career & Achievement*, The Hatherleigh Company, Ltd.

fer the company of other children most of the time? Did we do particularly well writing essays in school, or were we better at biology? Given a choice of summer jobs, did we like to sell merchandise in a department store, mow lawns, or coach sports at a camp?

The more the responsibilities of our work today afford us an outlet for the talents and interests we had as children, then the more effective and fulfilled we can be in it.

In recent years, it seems that people of all ages have been having difficulty focusing their energies. Sometimes they have focused adequately, but followed the Pied Piper of contemporary mores down the path to confusion, disillusionment, and disappointment. Ironically, the brighter and more creative they are, the more of a problem they seem to have. It's hard to commit yourself to organizations that are as enormous as many of our society's corporations have become. Studies have shown that when an organization becomes a certain size, it is difficult for most people within it to identify with the whole. Automatically, they see themselves as part of a smaller segment; these segments multiply and become more self-contained as the organization expands. We don't work for ABC Electronics; we work for the southwestern regional marketing division for product X that happens to be a part of ABC Electronics. Even within our own small department, we may never have an overall vision of what we are about. As a result, it is difficult to derive a sense of identity, purpose, and effectiveness from our jobs.

It's also difficult to commit ourselves to something that may well not survive. There has been a shift in our economy from heavy industry to technology, and many basic labor skills have rapidly become obsolete as new time-saving and money-saving devices have been introduced. Economies have become internationalized. Millions of workers have already had to face the need for retraining—a not-so-easy process that involves unlearning and relearning—and have been forced to uproot and relocate themselves and their families in order to survive. Once-rich corporations have gone bankrupt; many small, once-familiar companies have been acquired by large ones and disappeared.

The odds are stacked against our working within a given structure for the rest of our lives. If we begin working for ABC Electronics in our 20s, the company and its management may not even exist by the time we reach 35. And even if it lasts for a hundred years, our sense of loyalty is not likely to endure (if it was ever there in the first place). Ambition, opportunity, and change itself will probably lure us elsewhere.

Perhaps then, in some instances, this hesitancy to commit and the desire to keep options open really reflects an intuitively smart and uniquely creative approach to a most uncertain future and the determination to be ready for it when it comes.

"Of course," says Dr. Flach, "such issues as keeping a roof over our heads and food on the table don't disappear. What is called for is the creative ability to live on more than one level at a time, finding a place for oneself within the existing system to the degree that this is necessary for day-to-day survival, yet remaining somewhat apart, open to change within ourselves and our world. To accomplish this requires resilience and, as part of resilience, the discovery of a meaning that will give purpose to our lives."

**CRUNCH FITNESS**

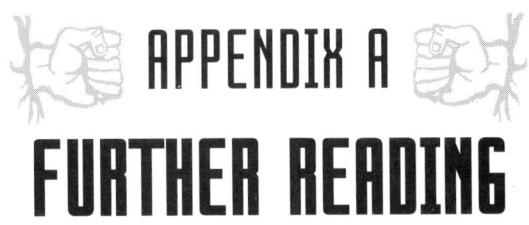

# APPENDIX A
# FURTHER READING

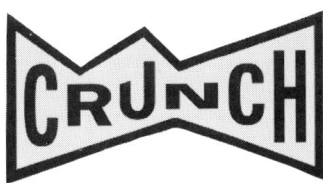

## NO TIME TO READ?

News flash: People today are under a constant barrage of information from television, newspapers, radio, and the Internet. Doctors have found, however, that this continual exposure to news reports contributes to stress. Give yourself a break: For one week, don't listen to the news and don't read the morning newspaper. You'll survive, trust me.

Escape with a good novel or biography. Or read other books about how to tame stress and workaholism. The following books are recommended on the Web site of Workaholics Anonymous, www.ai.mit.edu/people/wa/home.html. Check your local library if any of the books you are interested in are out of print.

Chained to the Desk: A Guidebook for Workaholics, Their Partners and Children, and the Clinicians Who Treat Them, Bryan E. Robinson, New York University Press, 1998.

Climb a Fallen Ladder: How to Survive in a Downsized America, Rochelle H. Gordon, M.D., and Catherine E. Harold, Hatherleigh Press, 1997.

The End of Work: The Decline of the Global Labor Force and the Dawn of the Post-Market Era, Jeremy Rifkin, J.P. Putnam Sons, 1995.

Overdoing It: How to Slow Down and Take Care of Yourself, Bryan E. Robinson, Health Communications, Inc., 1992.

The Power of Being: For People Who Do Too Much, Christian R. Komor, Renegade House Productions, 1992.

Resilience: The Power to Bounce Back When the Going Gets Tough!, Frederich Flach, M.D., Hatherleigh Press, 1997.

Taming Your Gremlin: A Guide to Enjoying Yourself, Richard D. Carson, HarperPerennial, 1983.

When Work Doesn't Work Anymore, Perle McKenna, Delacorte, 1997.

Women & Anxiety, Helen DeRosis, M.D., Hatherleigh Press, 1998.

Work Addiction: Hidden Legacies of Adult Children, Bryan E. Robinson, Health Communications, Inc., 1989 (out of print).

Work Won't Love You Back: The Dual Career Couple's Survival Guide, Stevan E. Hobfoll and Ivonne H. Hobfoll, W.H. Freeman, 1994.

Workaholics: The Respectable Addicts, A Family Survival Guide, Barbara Killinger, Simon & Schuster, 1991.

Working, Studs Turkel, Random House, 1974.

Working Ourselves to Death: The High Cost of Workaholism and the Rewards of Recovery, Diane Fassel, HarperCollins Publishers, 1990 (out of print).

# APPENDIX B
# ADVANCED WORKOUTS

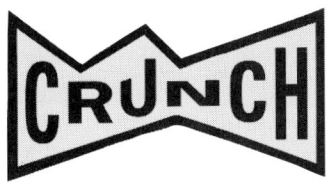

When the workouts described earlier in this book are no longer challenging, try these advanced workouts. You still need to use the clock, but you will take a much shorter rest between exercises. You may also want to use a heart rate monitor to make sure you're maintaining your heart rate at a higher level.

The jump rope will play a key role in everything you do. Where you had a break time in the previous workouts, now you will jump rope instead! This will keep your heart rate up and keep you sweating.

### Advanced Office Workout

To keep the office workout challenging, jump rope in between every set instead of resting. Instead of doing five minutes of one-leg squats, do 15 one-leg squats. Also, add more push-ups and crunches and use a heavier body bar.

### Advanced Business Travel Workout

To take the business travel workout to the next level, jump rope for speed during the 10 minutes and increase the reps from 15 to 25.

## THE WORKAHOLIC'S WORKOUT

## THE ADVANCED GYM WORKOUT

### CHEST

| Reps/time | Exercise |
|---|---|
| 8 minutes | warm up on stationary bike |
| 15 reps | bench press |
| 15 reps | dumbbell flies |
| 25 reps | push-ups |
| 5 minutes | jump rope |

The above chest exercises should take the chest muscles, along with the triceps and shoulders, to total fatigue. In terms of weights, you should start out lifting 75% of your one max* rep on the bench and anywhere from 15 to 40-lb. dumbbells for the flies, depending on how strong you are.

### BACK

| Reps/time | Exercise |
|---|---|
| 75% of max. | seated cable row |
| 75% of max. | lat pull-downs |
| 75% of max. | pull-ups |
| 5 minutes | jump rope |

### LEGS

| Reps/time | Exercise |
|---|---|
| 15 reps | squats with body bar, using with 60% max. weight |
| 15 reps | leg extensions |
| 15 reps | leg curls |
| 5 minutes | jump rope |

This workout is rigorous on the body. You can work out any two body parts in the same day, but never the same body parts two days in a row.

To keep challenging yourself:

1. increase the percentage of your max.
2. jump rope faster each time, keeping your heart rate up about 75 to 80% of your max. heart rate.

*Max refers to the weight you can lift only once (i.e., for one rep of the exercise).

# CRUNCH FITNESS

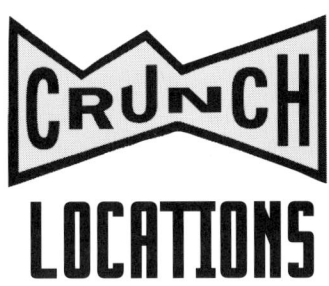

# LOCATIONS

Where to work out, pretend to work out, or just stand around calling our personal trainers "Hans" and "Franz" under your breath.

## NEW YORK CITY

404 Lafayette Street
(Astor Place and 4th Avenue)
212.614.0120

54 East 13th Street
(University and Broadway)
212.475.2018

162 West 83rd Street
(Columbus and Amsterdam)
212.875.1902

623 Broadway (at Houston)
212.420.0507

152 Christopher Street
(at Greenwich Street)
212.366.3725

1109 Second Avenue
(at 59th Street)
212.758.3434

144 W. 38th St.
(7th Ave. & Broadway)
212.869.7788

## LOS ANGELES

8000 Sunset Blvd.
(West Hollywood)
323.654.4550

## SAN FRANCISCO

1000 Van Ness Avenue
(Geary and O'Farrell)
415.931.1100

## MISSION VIEJO

The Kaleidoscope Center
27741 Crown Valley Parkway
949.582.8181

## MIAMI

1259 Washington Avenue
(South Beach)
305.674.8222

## CRUNCH LOCATIONS

### ATLANTA AREA
### [ALL LOCATIONS: 800.660.5433]

Crunch Club Cobb
North by NW Office Park
1775 Water Place
Atlanta, GA 30339

Crunch Roswell
Roswell Exchange
11060 Alpharetta Highway
Roswell, GA 30076

Crunch Gwinnett
Gwinnett Prado
2300 Pleasant Hill Road
Duluth, GA 30136

Crunch Buckhead
3365 Piedmont Road, Suite 1010
Atlanta, GA

Crunch Town Center
Main Street Shopping Center
2600 Prado Lane
Marietta, GA 30066

Crunch Stone Mountain
Stone Mountain Square
5370 Highway 78 South
Stone Mountain, GA 30087

### CHICAGO

Crunch Chicago
350 North State Street
Chicago, IL 60610
312.527.8100

### TOKYO

Crunch Omotesando
4-3-24 Jingumae Sibuya

Coming soon to Las Vegas!

Visit us on the Web at
www.crunch.com

## CRUNCH FITNESS

# Have questions about this workout?

### Ask the authors at:
# WWW.GETFITNOW.COM
*The **hottest** fitness spot on the internet!*

FEATURING...

"Ask the Expert" Q&A Boards

Stimulating Discussion groups

Cool Links

Great Photos

Full-Motion Videos

Downloads

The Five Star Fitness Team

Hot Product Reviews

And More!

**Log on today to receive a FREE catalog or call us at**
**1-800-906-1234**

## Personal Training Coupon

### 15% OFF! 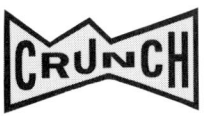 15% OFF!

IT'S EASY... Come into any CRUNCH location and receive 15% off your first purchase of personal training. Then just sign, date, and present this coupon at the fitness desk to set up your session.

_____     _____
MEMBER NAME                                                    SIGNATURE

_____     _____
TRAINER NAME                                                   TRAINER SIGNATURE

_____
DATE OF SESSION

Cannot be combined with any other offer. Valid for one use only

- - - - - - - - - - - CUT AT DOTTED LINE - - - - - - - - - - -

### GUEST PASS

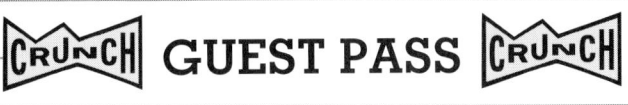

### $22 value!

Must show picture ID to use facility.
The same guest may use only two guest passes per year

_____     _____
MEMBERSHIP REP                                                 EXPIRATION DATE

### OUR MISSION AND PHILOSOPHY

We at CRUNCH warmly welcome people from all walks of life,
regardless of shape, size, sex, or ability.
People don't have to be flawless to feel at home at CRUNCH. We don't care
if our members are 18 or 80, fat or thin, short or tall, muscular or mushy, blond or bald,
or anywhere in between. CRUNCH is not competitive, it is non-judgmental,
it is not elitist, it does not represent a kind of person.
CRUNCH is a gym; a movement which is growing as we continue to perfect our ability
to create an environment where our members don't feel self-conscious,
and don't worry about what others think.
At the heart of CRUNCH's core stands a tremendously experienced and energetic staff
dedicated to creating an environment where everyone feels accepted—
a truly unique place!

### WWW.CRUNCH.COM
The **hottest** fitness spot on the internet!

## OUR MISSION AND PHILOSOPHY

We at CRUNCH warmly welcome people from all walks of life,
regardless of shape, size, sex, or ability.
People don't have to be flawless to feel at home at CRUNCH. We don't care
if our members are 18 or 80, fat or thin, short or tall, muscular or mushy, blond or bald,
or anywhere in between. CRUNCH is not competitive, it is non-judgmental,
it is not elitist, it does not represent a kind of person.
CRUNCH is a gym; a movement which is growing as we continue to perfect our ability
to create an environment where our members don't feel self-conscious,
and don't worry about what others think.
At the heart of CRUNCH's core stands a tremendously experienced and energetic staff
dedicated to creating an environment where everyone feels accepted—
a truly unique place!

# WWW.CRUNCH.COM

*The **hottest** fitness spot on the internet!*

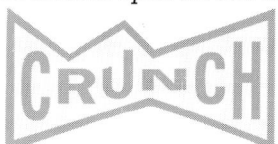

------- CUT AT DOTTED LINE -------

### NEW YORK CITY
404 Lafayette Street
(Astor Place and 4th Street)
212.614.0120

54 East 13th Street
(University and Broadway)
212.475.2018

162 West 83rd Street
(Columbus and Amsterdam)
212.875.1902

623 Broadway (at Houston)
212.420.0507

152 Christopher Street
(at Greenwich Street)
212.366.3725

1109 Second Avenue
(at 59th Street)
212.758.3434

144 W. 38th St.
(7th Ave. & Broadway)
212.869.7788

### LOS ANGELES
8000 Sunset Blvd.
(West Hollywood)
323.654.4550

### SAN FRANCISCO
1000 Van Ness Avenue
(Geary and O'Farrell)
415.931.1100

### MISSION VIEJO
The Kaleidoscope Center
27741 Crown Valley
  Parkway
949.582.8181

### MIAMI
1259 Washington Avenue
(South Beach)
305.674.8222

### ATLANTA AREA
(All locations: 800.660.5433)

Crunch Club Cobb
North by NW Office Park
1775 Water Place
Atlanta, GA 30339

Crunch Gwinnett
Gwinnett Prado
2300 Pleasant Hill Road
Duluth, GA 30136

Crunch Town Center
Main Street Shopping
  Center
2600 Prado Lane
Marietta, GA 30066

Crunch Roswell
Roswell Exchange
11060 Alpharetta Highway
Roswell, GA 30076

Crunch Buckhead
3365 Piedmont Road,
Suite 1010
Atlanta, GA

Crunch Stone Mountain
Stone Mountain Square
5370 Highway 78 South
Stone Mountain, GA 30087

### CHICAGO
Crunch Chicago
350 North State Street
Chicago, IL 60610
312.527.8100

**LAS VEGAS COMING SOON!**

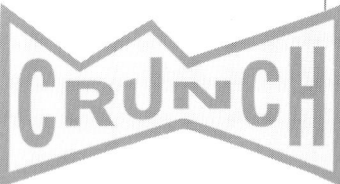